Battles of
Life and Death

Battles of
Life and Death

David Hellerstein

1986

HOUGHTON MIFFLIN COMPANY BOSTON

Library of Congress Cataloging in Publication Data

Hellerstein, David.
Battles of life and death.

1. Hellerstein, David.   2. Medical students —
United States — Biography.   3. Interns (Medicine) —
United States — Biography.   4. Residents (Medicine) —
United States — Biography.   5. Physician and patient.
I. Title.
RI54.H337A33   1986   610'.7'1173   [B]   85-24941
ISBN 0-395-40459-2

Printed in the United States of America

S   10   9   8   7   6   5   4   3   2   1

The author is grateful for permission to quote from "The Last Words of My English Grandmother," from *Selected Poems* by William Carlos Williams. Copyright © 1962 by William Carlos Williams. Reprinted by permission of New Directions Publishing Corporation.

The essays in this collection first appeared in the following publications: "A Death in the Glitter Palace," "Fire in the Hills," "Children of the Valley," "Related Illnesses," "The Gray Ones," "The Madonna of Red Hook," "The Electric Prince," "Beds," "The Assistant," and "Studies of the Heart" in the *North American Review;* "The Battle for the Dead" and "Witnesses" (original title, "The Heat") in *Esquire;* "Touching" (original title, "The Training of a Gynecologist") in *Ms.*

The identities of the people described in these essays and the circumstances by which they could be identified have been changed in order to ensure privacy.

To my parents

ACKNOWLEDGMENTS

I would like to gratefully acknowledge the help of my editors, including Robley Wilson, Jr., Marilyn Johnson, Betsy Carter, Ellen Fair, Nan Talese, and Signe Warner; my teacher, the late Robert Fitzgerald; the MacDowell Colony, for the time and creative solitude necessary to complete this work; and especially, for her support and understanding during these long years of dual apprenticeship, my wife, Lisa Perry Hellerstein.

CONTENTS

Introduction

WHEN I CAME into the Intensive Care Unit, Mr. Peraldi turned his face to the wall. They'd just extubated him, and you could see the marks of adhesive tape around his mouth. When he finally said something it was in a hoarse, raw voice. "Go away." He was middle aged, balding and full of fury. Half a dozen IV bottles hung overhead, the tubing from which dove through the skin of his neck. Monitors blinked on the wall, and a bag of urine hung at the foot of the bed. Diligent medical student that I was, I persisted for half an hour, holding stethoscope to his side and palpating and percussing though his hands pushed me away, asking question after question without response. Finally I left the bedside. At the nurses' station, a woman stopped me.

She was Mr. Peraldi's friend, she said nervously; she'd found him lying unconscious on his living room floor. He'd been horribly depressed recently, in trouble at work. A week ago he'd stopped his insulin shots and waited calmly, blood sugar rising, until he slipped into a coma. He's so *depressed*, she told me, he wants to die.

In my consult note (that month I was representing Endocrinology) I wrote that, besides the obvious hyperosmolar nonketotic state, the patient seemed depressed, even suicidal; he should be observed closely; a Psychiatry consultant should be called in. Not bad, I thought — a thorough evaluation, looking at the whole patient, the way we were always taught was so important. I went away very pleased with myself. On rounds, though, the Endocrine fellow, four years my senior, scowled at my note. Beside my diagnosis of depression he wrote in capitals: DISAGREE!

"What do you mean?" I said.

The fellow explained. Our professor thought psychiatry was bunk. Whenever he saw a note like this one, the professor would explode, denouncing not only psychiatry but whoever had been unlucky enough to write such nonsense. The best thing to do was to tear up my note and write another one.

"What should I say caused the coma?" I asked.

"Brittle diabetes," said the fellow.

"Brittle? There's nothing brittle about it. He took his insulin regularly for years. It was only when he stopped his shots . . ."

It was futile. The fellow was unmoved. He saw my point, but his advice remained the same.

I thought awhile. The medical record was a legal document, a scientific record as well. My note was already part of the chart. On the other hand, I was just beginning the clerkship, and I was considering applying for residency at this hospital — and it just wouldn't bode well to get off to a bad start.

Just before the professor came by for afternoon rounds, I rewrote my note from beginning to end, without mentioning depression or suicide — or psychiatry, the field I myself would enter one year hence.

I have no idea what happened to Mr. Peraldi — nothing bad, I hope — but what has returned whenever I think about that incident is a jolt of alarm, a sense of disbelief. Alarm not only at the professor, whose prejudices might endanger his patients, but at the power of fearful anticipation, which could cause a scientifically minded fellow to veer sharply from truth and cause me, an eager medical student, to resort to dishonesty in a potentially dangerous situation.

More than that, the jolt came because I thought I already *knew* medicine — how one worked at the bedside, how one conferred with colleagues in a nurses' station, how one prescribed and examined and counseled and interpreted equivocal lab results. The incident with Mr. Peraldi was only one of a hundred incidents in a decade of medical training in California and Boston and New York that were to shake certainties accumulated during a childhood in one of the most medical of families.

Four generations of my family have been doctors. My maternal great-grandfather was a general practitioner in Cleveland; my maternal grandfather was one of the earliest cardiologists; my mother is a pediatrician; my father is a cardiologist and professor of medicine; and the rest of the family, from biochemist and pathologist uncles to aunts in nursing and social work to cousins and siblings in medicine and surgery, has ramified its various branches and roots through the rich soil of the medical professions. Even my earliest memory is that of a bedside visit — being lowered, at the age of one and a half or two, onto the starchy white sheets of my grandfather Hellerstein's hospital bed, where he lay, having been run down by a drunk driver, and where a few days later he died.

From the age of five or six I accompanied my father to University Hospital on rounds, where he'd leave me in the nurses' station or occasionally take me with him and hoist me up on patients' beds so I could listen to their hearts. At eight I could read electrocardiograms in a rudimentary way and hear the swish of a murmur. At eleven I moved to my father's attic study, where coils of electrocardiogram tape and wooden boxes of lantern slides and stacks of medical journals surrounded me. The bedside lamp, a present to my father from his students, had a shade that was inked with the black squiggles of the heart's QRS complex. When bored, I paged through medical books, from *Surgical Pathology* to *Symposia in Cardiology* to my favorite, *Diseases of Women*. On the shelves around my bedroom window my father had arranged a collection of hearts, real *human* hearts some of them. They were preserved in sparkling Lucite blocks, or in sticky yellow wax that came off on your fingers, their ventricles cut open to show calcified valves.

Sometimes my brothers and I would drive with our father from Cleveland to Canton or Sandusky, Ohio, where he went to see a difficult case the local doctors couldn't figure out; other times we'd accompany him to the site of his cardiology and occupational health research projects — a firehouse, a parachuting field. And late at night, I'd come down for a snack and find my father in the yellow breakfast room, which had a map of the world on one wall, going over spread-out EKGs, and he'd show me the poor R-wave progression and inverted T waves of sick hearts. And always, at home, the phone would be ringing. Is Dr. Hellerstein there? the caller would ask. Which one, we'd reply, our father or our mother? We'd calmly take urgent messages. Mr. Wright is having chest pain. The Kestlebaums' baby has a temp of 104 degrees. The resident on call has a question. We even helped our father do surgery on the family dog, removing big stony tumors from under his skin and suturing him up.

On birthdays and holidays the extended family would gather at my grandparents' house. The doctors would all gather around the dining room table, and, in low voices, talk about the new diuretic that had just come out, or about the Academy of Medicine, or hospital politics. Now that Pritchard's taking over the department . . . , they would say. Or, What about that new fellow they've got from Pittsburgh? Or, The house officers don't seem very happy this year . . .

I thought I knew medicine backward and forward.

Yet, entering medical school, and particularly on my first rotations in the hospital, I ran into one baffling surprise after another, enough jolts and shocks to set my head spinning.

For one thing, there was so much I didn't know. The bits of cardiology I had acquired through osmosis represented only a small corner of medicine. There were all the basic sciences — histology and biochemistry and anatomy and pathology. There were innumerable diseases whose existence I'd never suspected — leukemias, lymphomas, diabetes, nephroses, psychoses, autoimmune disorders. There were drugs and radiological procedures and types of surgery I'd never heard of, and everything under the sun had its indications, contraindications, side effects, interactions, complications. Hundreds of chemical tests could be ordered for blood or urine or spinal fluid or just about any liquid that could be drained or squeezed or otherwise coaxed out of the human body.

Through medical school I was in a state of perpetual amazement, dazzled by this white stream of unending, infinitely complex knowledge. It was a shock to find how technical medicine was. The intricate procedures of resuscitating the heart attack victim, or quenching the leukemic's blue flame of fever — one could stand for hours in rounds, talking about potassium and bicarbonate, about the A-V O_2 gradient, the ventilation-perfusion abnormality, the metabolic alkalosis compensated by a respiratory acidosis, and when it was all over you were half convinced you were talking about a complex chemical solution, not a sick human being. Distressingly much of the disease one encountered in the high-technology hospital setting was actually caused by previous treatment.

I found the actual minute-to-minute work of medicine was rarely glorious, usually incredibly mundane. You could be completely exhausted after losing only two or three hours of sleep, not even enough to brag about. There were so many phone calls to make to track down lost lab tests. You were constantly scrawling something, whether on order sheets or progress note paper or prescription pads or insurance forms. The hardest things had nothing to do with your special knowledge — it could be unbelievably difficult to soothe an anxious relative or just to get a patient to take his pills regularly. And I found it surprisingly draining to comfort, to calm, to give support when I was feeling exhausted and overwhelmed myself.

But my biggest surprise in medical training was how strange *I* was. I was fascinated by the interactions between doctor and patient, by the reality of what happened at the bedside and how different it was from what you read in medical texts. The talk, the actual words used to convince a family to give consent for autopsy of their dead father or husband intrigued me but didn't seem to interest my colleagues much. Negotiations undertaken when you tried to draw blood from a sick child rivaled the Paris peace talks. A patient dying of leukemia experienced a range of emotions — expectation, disappointment, closeness, frightening distance — that was as great and baffling as anything I'd ever seen on the stage. There were odd incongruities: highly skilled doctors seemed unable to adequately treat the pain of their burn patients, usually compassionate residents avoided talking to dying patients on rounds. These facts captured my attention as much as the silent biochemical reactions of the human body.

I always assumed I would end up a cardiologist, like my

father and grandfather, if only through having a twenty-year head start on my medical school classmates. I assumed, too, that if I had creative talents they would take shape in the research laboratory and that, like my father and grandfather before me, I would end up investigating myocardial function. Yet the passion for research, which animated them both, was curiously lacking in me, or, if present, it had been transmuted to a radically different form. As I went through medical school I also began to write. And I emerged not as a cardiologist and researcher but as a psychiatrist and writer.

Psychiatry, as I discovered during residency training, is even odder than medicine. In medicine you can at least see the spots on the skin or the X-ray shadow of a tumor on the lung, but in psychiatry you truly appreciate the patient's problem by living it. An internist can keep a safe clinical distance. But even in this age of PET scanners and neuroendocrine tests and psychotropic drugs, a psychiatrist lives in the realm of the emotions. Psychiatry requires that you think so differently from other medical specialists that you practically have to unlearn all the attitudes and instincts you so painfully acquired in medical school and internship. The reflexes of quickness, of definitive action, must give way to silence, to patience with ambiguity; facts give way to feelings. But for all its bafflements I have found psychiatry more interesting, more congenial, less rigidly technical than medicine, and more challenging, because of the extreme difficulty of learning to listen deeply.

But in one way both medicine and psychiatry are alike: they are both in crisis as this century draws to a close. Both are threatened by changes in financial reimbursement, by inequities in supply and demand, by cutbacks in research moneys; both are increasingly hemmed in by new legislation. And both increasingly hear complaints from their consumers, who feel cheated by a science that promises more than it delivers, by practitioners who are often described as being hurried and impersonal.

Patients often write about their experiences; doctors, trained in silence, rarely do. However, by writing about a world that is commonly misunderstood and misrepresented, one can show the realities of life better than through a thousand surveys or questionnaires. A doctor who writes can complete the picture, can show not only the extent of problems and miscommunications between doctor and patient, the paradoxes, the confusions and incongruities along with the victories and small miracles, but can also open the possibility of finding solutions.

A Death in
the Glitter Palace

I

EVEN NOW, more than five years after her death, I cannot entirely get Cha Nan Chen out of my mind. She was not family or a lover, this twenty-eight-year-old Vietnamese woman with a flat, broad face and two lethal diseases racing to kill her, but instead a patient of mine, to whom I struggled to give good care under hopeless circumstances. With Cha Nan Chen I shared the doctor's distant intimacy, even when I ordered the shots of morphine that let her die.

Her first malignancy, Hodgkin's disease, a tumor of lymph nodes, had been cured by the time she came to the Medicine 3 Oncology Team at a major university medical center, where I, as a fourth-year student, was doing an advanced rotation. A combination of cell poisons and radiation therapy had melted it away. In its place, whether as a result of therapy or as an ironic natural evolution, mutant cells of acute myelogenous leukemia (AML) began colonizing her decimated bone marrow and clogging her blood vessels. She had traded a cancer of the lymph nodes, with expected survival of perhaps three or four years, for a cancer of the blood cells, which killed her in thirty days. The rationalization that such complications are uncommon, occurring in perhaps 5 percent of cases, and that the lifespan of cancer patients given such aggressive therapy is, on the average, lengthened, gives comfort only to the statistician. But Cha Nan Chen was my patient and I mourn her.

A physician writing in the *New England Journal of Medicine* that year described the problem dispassionately:

> An increasing incidence of therapy-linked Acute Myelogenous Leukemia is being reported in patients who receive chemotherapy, radiation therapy or immunosuppressive drugs for neoplastic and non-neoplastic diseases, including Hodgkin's Disease, lymphoma, ovarian carcinoma and others. The response rate of these patients to chemotherapy is poor, with remission rates of less than 10 percent in most series.

Or, as Susan Sontag wrote more succinctly in *Illness as Metaphor,* "The treatment meant to cure kills." The radiation and the poisonous drugs given to cancer patients, especially in combination, have a distressing tendency to create new, incurable disease. Cha Nan Chen had received both chemotherapy and radiation. Though I did not know it at the time, when she came to be my patient it was too late: she was as good as dead.

The young Vietnamese woman of Chinese extraction came to our clinic in March of 1979. For the past three weeks she had felt tired and lethargic, and small red dots by the dozen had appeared on her lower legs, upper chest and back. A few days before, while shopping with her three-year-old daughter and her father, who had recently arrived from Vietnam via Hong Kong, she began coughing and shaking uncontrollably. At home, despite aspirin and cold washcloths to her forehead and chest, she burned with fever for a night and a day. In the clinic, she saw the doctor who had been following her progress after treatment for Hodgkin's disease. He had blood drawn, which, under the microscope, revealed a frightening scarcity of white blood cells and platelets. Even more disturbing, among the white corpuscles of her blood were peculiarly "young" forms, cells that normally are confined to the marrow until further development has occurred. He telephoned the Med 3 resident, Larry, who sent me, his subintern, down to clinic to admit the patient.

Oncology is a star department in the glitter palace medicine of the university; unlike Pediatrics or Obstetrics, which attract the young and insolvent, Oncology counts among its patients professionals and businessmen and others whom large amounts of savings have not protected against malignancy. The clinic, located in the hospital basement, is luxuriously carpeted and wallpapered, all color coordinated, and trays of fruit are provided for clinic physicians. Sitting in the Conference Room, I munched grapes while reviewing the new patient's records.

Two thick manila volumes told me that three years ago this young woman, a recent immigrant to the United States, had been swept with inexplicable fevers that came and went without cause. At night she would wake, drenched in sweat. And though she did not notice them at first, rubber-hard bumps — lymph nodes — swelled in her neck. Her doctor did notice them, waited a while to see if they would disappear, and when they did not, sent her to a surgeon who sliced one out. A pathologist "elsewhere" (as one refers to hospitals outside the academic medical center "here") saw whorls of crazily proliferating cells, and diagnosed Hodgkin's disease of the nodular sclerosing type. One of four types of the disease, having intermediate mortality, it's worse than lymphocyte predominant but nowhere near as lethal as lymphocyte depletion. She was sent "here," where similar hard nodes were noted in the folds of her groin, and a hard, enlarged spleen, grown down below the margin of her left ribs, was discovered through abdominal palpation.

Then the efficient machinery of the medical center's Hodgkin's disease protocol was set into motion. It is a marvel of glitter palace medicine: costly, scientific, aggressive, requiring the cooperation of half a dozen different departments within the medical center, and achieving heretofore unexcelled results in the treatment of rare disease. Patients with Hodgkin's disease flock to the area for treatment, much as prospective heart transplant recipients, drowning in the fluids of their own hearts' failure, wait in motel rooms and apartments up and down the strip for motorcyclists to smash their brains out on California highways and provide new hearts for them.

Along with routine blood studies, chest X rays and so forth, another node, from the young woman's groin, was taken for biopsy, which confirmed the findings in her neck. She underwent a bone biopsy and a lymphangiogram, in which dye is injected into the tiny lymph vessels of the feet to illuminate to X ray the lymph nodes that enwrap the descending aorta. Then she was sliced wide open by surgeons who removed her spleen and took biopsies of her liver and abdominal cavity nodes to detect the spread of disease. This process of "staging" showed disease in her spleen, but not in her liver or bone. Her disease fit category PS-III-SB, pathological stage III disease (*S,* involving the spleen, and *B,* meaning symptomatic in onset), and she was recommended for a combination of chemotherapy and radiotherapy. Radiotherapy came first: total nodal irradiation (TNI), which consisted of large doses of X rays to an area of her body from neck to groin, a "mantle" of lymph node–bearing regions of her neck and chest, and an "inverted

Y" from belly to hips. Her heart and lungs and ovaries were protected from the decimating radiation by "shields." All this Cha Nan Chen tolerated well, or so I gathered from the records, as she did the ensuing chemotherapy, eight monthly courses of Bleo-MOPP, a combination of five drugs it was hoped would be more poisonous to the cancer than to the patient. All treatment had ended in October 1976. Since then she had been well. The Oncology Clinic flow sheet listed her monthly blood counts, which were stable, and each visit's chest X ray, weight and vital signs, showing no change. Until three weeks ago, Cha Nan Chen had been, in Oncology jargon, NED, that is, with no evidence of disease — a glitter palace cure.

The woman I saw lying on a clinic examining table was young, Oriental, with a broad and not particularly pretty face to which sweat had plastered strands of black hair. She wore a hospital gown and cheap clunky shoes, and she had wrapped her arms around herself to lessen her shaking and terror. I introduced myself.

"Why do I have to be in the hospital again? Why do I have to be sick?"

I was afraid she'd start crying. I stood awkwardly beside her, waiting for her to regain her composure.

"I am sorry," she said. "What do you want to know?"

I questioned her about the Hodgkin's and its cure and her new symptoms, then examined her, noticing the red spots like scattered flecks of blood across her back, down her chest almost to her breasts, along her shins. The roof of her mouth, too, was scattered with them. My stethoscope against her clammy back transmitted the dry rubbings of collapsed lung. And her abdomen, though scarred with surgery and burned with a permanent radiation tan, showed no clues to disease.

She wanted to know what I'd found.

"Well, red spots, of course," I said. "And you're hot, feverish, and you have a cough. I think you will have to be hospitalized."

"Oh," she said, looking down at her clunky shoes, absolutely desolate.

"But we'll try to get you home as soon as possible."

Later that afternoon, I was standing by the nurses' station, finishing my note on Cha Nan, when Larry, my resident, returned. He was supposed to supervise my every move but often disappeared for hours at a time, off running in the hills or weight lifting or eating dinner with his girlfriend. Short and top-heavy with muscle, Larry leaned up against me to read my note.

28 y.o. ♀ NSHD CSIISB/PSIIISB 3 yr. hx., s/p TNI 4500 rads mantle/3500 rads inverted Y, last 4/76, s/p Bleo-MOPP, last 10/76 → now 3 wks. hx. fatigue, cough & fever, blasts on smear → ?? 2° AML

He borrowed my stethoscope and lumbered off, thick-necked as a Minotaur, to examine her. Twenty minutes later he returned, slapping the stethoscope against his thigh.

"So you think it's AML?" he said.

"The smear sure looked like it. Blasts all over. I've got it here, in my pocket, if you want to see it."

He shrugged. "What have you done so far?"

"Cultured everything — blood, sputum, urine, throat. Chest X ray. All the usual bloods. Reverse isolation. Six units of platelets. Oh, also, I wrote for a Hematology consult and scheduled a marrow for tomorrow. I didn't know whether to write for K, G and C."

"Let's wait on the antibiotics," he suggested. "Now, what do you want to do with her?"

"What do you mean? Treat her. Find out where the infection is —"

"No, no, I mean the AML."

"I . . . I don't know. If it *is* AML, I guess, induce her. She's got a three-year-old daughter, she wants to get home to her."

"They don't respond, these AMLs, to induction like the virgin ones do," he said. "Probably just end up killing her."

"The AML definitely will," I said. "She's already bleeding, febrile, probably septic. What choice do we have?"

"She's your patient."

The next morning, Cha Nan, lying on her belly, her flank scrubbed with iodine solution, draped with blue towels, anesthetized as well as can be done with Xylocaine, screamed as I screwed a hollow metal bit into the bone of her hip. The bone marrow is one of medicine's most barbaric procedures, the exact technique one uses to drill a core from a tree to determine its age, at which one is most successful if speedy as a Civil War surgeon amputating a leg with only his sharp saw and bottle of whiskey. My technique, though, lacking both brutality and speed, was immensely more painful. I could make her neither maple tree nor soldier; instead, she remained a weeping Vietnamese woman who had lost her homeland and whose husband, an American veteran, had deserted her in the first illness, who was succumbing now to a second and worse disease we doctors had given her. Trembling, I screwed metal into bone. She writhed. I attached a syringe, tried to suck out marrow. She screamed. No marrow. "Just get the core," said Larry. I was drenched in sweat. I unscrewed the needle, hoping a red core of bone and marrow would stay caught in its hollow center. But no — empty. "Have to do it again," said Larry. "We *need* the core." I stepped away from the bed, tore off my gloves. My bare hands shook. "I can't. You do it." Larry rolled up his sleeves, showing a weight lifter's biceps, triceps, deltoids; he snapped on a pair of gloves and began.

Later, still sweating, I said, "I don't know *why* . . . I've done it half a dozen times before . . . I just couldn't . . . couldn't get the *distance* right."

He said, "You have to get *on* the bed, then bear down with every ounce of your weight."

We ordered fresh frozen plasma and six units of platelets to help her clotting, but when I left at nine that night, and indeed, when I arrived the next morning, the bone marrow site in her hip was still oozing blood.

I I

> Treatment [of cancer] . . . has a military flavor. Radiotherapy uses the metaphors of aerial warfare; patients are "bombarded" with toxic rays. And chemotherapy is chemical warfare, using poisons. Treatment aims to "kill" cancer cells (without, it is hoped, killing the patient). Unpleasant side effects of treatment are advertised, indeed overadvertised. ("The agony of chemotherapy" is a standard phrase.) It is impossible to avoid damaging or destroying healthy cells . . . but it is thought that nearly any damage to the body is justified if it saves the patient's life. Often, of course, it doesn't work. (As in: "We had to destroy Ben Suc in order to save it.") There is everything but the body count.
>
>   SUSAN SONTAG, *Illness as Metaphor*

There is, with AML, the blast count: how many malignant cells float through the blood, like mines in a harbor.

Over the next few days the Med 3 team had several discussions about Cha Nan Chen. She was no sicker than half a dozen other patients on the service, although she did continue to run high fevers, to bleed from the marrow site and from her vagina (though her period had ended ten days ago), and, late at night, to break out in strange rashes that could be controlled only with large doses of steroids. The two interns on the service complained that she kept them up all night. Her marrow biopsy was fixed and read; it was packed tight with blasts, myeloid type. Hematology came to consult on the question of whether, and how, to treat what we now knew for certain was acute myeloid leukemia. They told us that the ordinary patient with AML, if untreated, will die within two months; if "induced" by intensive chemotherapy, which essentially wipes out the patient's bone marrow to allow the "good" cells to repopulate the areas where malignant cells have been killed, the average patient may live a year or more. They emphasized what we already knew: Cha Nan was not a typical patient, and her disease was far less likely to respond. For treatment they recommended Ara-C and 6-TG, which are in the class of "antimetabolite" drugs. In addition, they noted, "The patient will need to be supported with red cell, platelet, and white cell transfusions through her period of aplasia." While her bombarded bone marrow was unable to produce normal blood cells, we had to replace them. At morning rounds, the Med 3 team, including our ward attending, Dr. Brown, the two interns, and Larry and I, discussed what to do.

Larry said he was with me; he wanted to treat her, especially since Hematology, despite the odds, wanted to go ahead. Dr. Brown, who had seen many of these patients in recent years, said, "I'm really not sure if it's worth it."

"But her white count's zero point seven with sixty blasts. She's not responding to antibiotics. Unless we do something," I added, "she'll be dead in a few weeks."

"I don't disagree with that," said Dr. Brown. "I'm just saying that in the past, no matter what we've done, we haven't had good responses."

"Maybe you just haven't tried hard enough," said Larry.

After rounds I went to see Cha Nan. She lay in bed, watching cartoons on the TV hanging from the wall. Her face was bloated. I put on a blue face mask, wiped my stethoscope with an alcohol swab and washed my hands before touching her. Listening to her lungs, I discovered a new area of consolidation just below her left shoulder blade.

"Say EEEEE," I said.

"AAAAAA."

"EEEEEE."

"AAAAAA."

Infection had settled in her lung. Depressed, I said nothing.

"I had a terrible night," she said. "I could not sleep at all."

"I know, Cha Nan. The interns keep complaining. You just get too many fevers."

"Why is that, David? And why do I always keep bleeding?"

I sat on the bed beside her, and we talked for an hour about the Ara-C and 6-TG and the white cell transfusions. She had seen Hematology yesterday, and accepted their recommendations without hesitation. "It is like last time," she said. "It will be hard to be treated but I have to do it."

"We do want to get you back to your daughter."

We talked about her daughter, Charlotte, who had been born in the United States a few years after she left Vietnam with her husband, just before the Hodgkin's was discovered. She described the chaos of Saigon: the bombs and the refugees; the courtyard of a French hotel where she had stayed, where prostitutes sat for hours under umbrella tables, ordering nothing; the panic when the last planes were leaving; and the difficulty in getting her father out of the country after the collapse. Even now his status in the United States was uncertain.

"I have to get out of the hospital next week," she said, "for one day only. To go to the courthouse downtown and get him papers — permanent residency papers."

"I don't think you'll be able to," I said. "But I'll write a letter, saying you can't leave the hospital, and asking if they can send the papers here. Okay?"

"Can you do that?" Her hand, damp and ill, touched mine momentarily, then pulled away. She said, "I should not touch you?"

"To protect you," I said.

Ara-C and 6-TG began. I was on call a few nights later when she got her first white blood cell transfusion. It was Passover, and I'd been invited to my sister's home for Seder, but I just couldn't get away. The interns wanted the night off, too. I ate dinner alone in the almost-deserted cafeteria, and everything seemed to be going well with Cha Nan — the usual fever, bleeding, cough, red spots, nothing more — when I went to bed around midnight. At 2:00 A.M. my phone rang. It was Maureen, the night nurse.

"I'm worried about Cha Nan. She's got a horrible rash all over her legs. And her temp's up."

"What to?"

"Forty-one four."

"Oh, God. What's that in real degrees?"

"Over one oh six . . . I don't know . . . It's off the scale."

I lay in bed in my green scrub suit, the *thrum* of the Pediatrics ICU air conditioner on the roof nearby vibrating my panic loose.

"I've started an alcohol sponge bath, cooling blanket, Tylenol —"

"Is . . . is she having trouble breathing?"

"No."

"Well," I said, relieved, "I'll be there in a minute. You might call Larry, too."

I put on shoes and white coat and stumbled down the ward, where, except for Cha Nan's, disease seemed to have abated this Passover night. Silent, empty except for the ward clerk with a cup of coffee, reading a newspaper. I recalled what an English grad student friend had asked. "Do you get a sense of things like Lewis Thomas describes, of a wonderful and complex order to life? Do you get a sense of astonishment?" I told him I hadn't felt that, only the horror of fighting decay on multiple fronts; and the occasional victory attained only partial, a matter of delay. "What is there but time?" I had answered him. "If you can give a person that . . ."

In her room, Cha Nan lay in agony. Her legs were covered with a red confluent rash — maculopapular and erythematous, my chart note would say — ugly, spreading, furious. She was coughing, sweating, holding her right side.

Maureen said, "Her right flank's started hurting all of a sudden. I don't know what it is."

I washed, masked up, overwhelmed by a vision of Cha Nan as battlefield — an image put into words by Sontag that I only later discovered — as our burned and blasted terrain, defoliated, napalmed, cratered. She coughed worse with the white cells, which "localize to the site of infection," clogging her lungs as they attacked the bugs within; she flared like an incendiary torch; she shivered uncontrollably; her flank was sprayed with fire. She had sprouted, I noticed now, viral ulcers on her mouth. Herpes — herpes encephalitis would be a miserable way to go. Better to die of any bacteria. I seemed to pull away from it all, to see her from a great distance. I thought of my father, a young soldier, a doctor, standing at the entrance of Bergen-Belsen on the eve of the concentration camp's liberation; the stacks of bodies he photographed; the tiny photographs I discovered in a rubberized canvas bag in the back corner of a desk drawer in the attic room of my Ohio childhood, photographs that awakened in me inexplicable memories of one war I had not experienced and the expectation of another coming, in which I would be a soldier.

"How are you doing, Cha Nan?"

"Not too good," she said. "Cold."

"You've given Benadryl, right?" I asked Maureen. She nodded. "A hundred of Solu-Medrol, then, that's what we want." Lateness buzzed in the air. "And for her side, Demerol, Dilaudid, whatever's ordered."

"I have to check this out with the resident," she said.

"Fine," I said. To Cha Nan, "I know this is terrible. But your blast count *is* coming down. I think we're . . . you're making progress."

I went upstairs, wondering if any stem cells were left. If not, she might be getting from our treatment a third disease, aplastic anemia, worse than Hodgkin's and worse even than AML. Lying in bed unable to sleep, I couldn't help thinking of a tune from the Haggadah, sung tonight, after a full, leisurely Passover meal.

> Then came the butcher and slaughtered the ox
> That drank the water
> That smothered the fire
> That burned the stick
> That beat the dog
> That killed the cat
> That ate the kid
> My father bought for two zuzim.
> Chad godya, chad godya.

I fell asleep hearing the tune, and worrying about Cha Nan.

Her blast count went down: 70, 50, 36, 27, 11, 4, 1 . . . then, one day, 0.

"No blasts, Cha Nan! I think we're winning!" Said through blue paper masks, our white coats tenting around her so she entirely disappeared, as half a dozen stethoscopes clattered together on her sweaty back. "Listen!" said Larry. I listened. "You hear that? A new pleural rub." Her blasts were down but so were all her white cells. You and I have five or ten thousand floating through our vessels, squeezing through the sinusoids of our spleens, crawling among our bodily organs. She had six hundred, four hundred, three hundred. And the platelets given her burst in her veins. Once it was half a million; now fifteen thousand was the best we could manage. She coughed more daily. On X ray a white haze took refuge in the back gutter of her right lung. Not even the triple antibiotics — acronymically K, G and C — made it disappear, made her, talking about her father, who was working illegally in the city making trousers, able to control the paroxysms of coughing. I felt helpless as a country doctor of the old days with his bleeding bowls and jars of leeches. Whenever I came in, Maureen or another nurse was trying to start an IV in Cha Nan's battered arms. Every vein stick hurt, and every new IV blew under the corrosion of K, G and C or of 6-TG and Ara-C. The blood we dripped in could not replace what oozed out. Cardiac surgeons came to try placing a central line so Cha Nan would not have to get stuck so often for bloods and IVs. But they failed. "Anomalous venous system," they wrote. "Will try other side next week." Cha Nan was always crying.

Then the husband showed up: a small, embarrassed-looking ex-GI with a pointy chin and the look of a ferret or a weasel surprised at his kill. And with him he brought Charlotte, the little girl. Charlotte had Cha Nan's black hair, and an exquisite timidity. Passing the room I would see her, mask in hand, climbing on Cha Nan's belly. The room, when I entered it, which was more and more rarely, smelled vaguely rotten from the food her husband brought. I wondered just where he had been all this time.

I avoided her. Elisabeth Kübler-Ross may have an expla-

nation for my conduct, in terms of an effort to minimize impending loss; all I know is that the second cycle of Ara-C
and 6-TG ended, and Cha Nan looked worse than ever, and
the Med 3 team made briefer and more perfunctory rounds
on her. And when alone, often I would just pass by the
room, rather than poke my head inside with the latest white
count or to ask about the letter for Cha Nan's father. I had
dictated it: "To whom it may concern: Cha Nan Chen is my
patient at the University Medical Center, with the diagnosis
of Acute Myelogenous Leukemia, and is unable to leave the
hospital . . ." Yet it had not arrived from Dictation. Somewhere on the way from telephone to typewriter to ward,
those words for the old Chinese man had disappeared.

And so had her cells. Everything stayed down: blasts, white
cells, red cells, platelets. I knew why I avoided her. There were
no stem cells left.

                              I I I

Now when I look back and try to unravel the events of those
despairing days, I find somewhat clearer patterns. But still,
fragments, confusions. The decision to treat her was, of course,
not mine. I had some limited say in it. But I took on the bur-
den for the whole Med 3 team and five consulting services as
my own. As if I were responsible not only for the failure of
her treatment but for the presence of her disease. I began to
have the horrible suspicion that we were shortening her life,
that our vigorous treatment was just killing her more quickly
than her disease itself. The anguish of seeing her every day
convinced me beyond suspicion, even beyond the facts. I
worked harder on my other patients: a nineteen-year-old kid
with testicular seminoma, a Mexican lady with ovarian cancer, a fifty-eight-year-old man who had sprayed asbestos in a

World War II shipyard and now had mesothelioma, an old Swede with cancer of the prostate, a Greek surgeon, Dr. Odysseus, with non-Hodgkin's lymphoma. All were ill; all but the nineteen-year-old would eventually die of their cancer, yet our work could give them something: time. But Cha Nan, no. And I avoided her.

Anyone who is sick or who treats sick patients today knows that the doctor is less often a curer than an odds player, trying to heal more disease than he causes. He is no longer the powerless observer; with the "big gun" antibiotics, anticancer drugs and so on, which often have horrific side effects, he is inevitably made part of the disease. The doctor must maintain composure both against the knowledge that every treatment is some degree Russian roulette, and against the patient's blind hope for cure. Each is dangerous. Insulin "saves" the diabetic from early death only to make crippled blind amputees on dialysis; phenothiazines alleviate schizophrenia but make some patients into writhing, wheelchair-bound freaks. Halothane for anesthesia, phenylbutazone for arthritis can kill your liver dead. There is no shortage of other examples for the cynical doctor, for the patient chary of treatment. The death of Cha Nan Chen is one small example of the paradox of medicine in twentieth-century America: the doctor's helpless retreat from the effects of his own therapeutic "armamentarium." It is no accident that, as Sontag says, "Recently the fight against cancer has sounded like a colonial war." When and how do you pull out? And what of the ensuing collapse?

It was a relief to let her die.

She told me first, one Saturday morning when I came in to find her feverish as usual, "David, I don't want any more."

"Hematology wants to try once more," I said. "With the Ara-C and 6-TG." Though silently I doubted whether they had even seen her. For in their note they recommended another bone marrow, too, "To assess our progress."

"*They* want," she said.

"They think that —"

"No."

The next day, the Med 3 team discussed her again, sitting in our conference room with her latest numbers up on the blackboard. Nobody had much to say.

"So we're pulling back?" I asked at the end.

Dr. Brown nodded. "She's finished," he said. "Up her morphine dose, stop her K, G and C, her blood products. If her IV falls out, keep it out. Agreed?"

Afterward I went to see her. At the foot of the bed sat her father, a shriveled Chinese with bushy gray hair. The letter that had gotten lost, that I had not dictated again, gnawed at me. Cha Nan's husband, unshaven, had the Sunday newspaper on his lap. Cha Nan lay in bed, eyes open only enough to show whites, and she breathed only every six or eight seconds, with shudders each time. Cheyne-Stokes respirations, a terminal pattern, evidence of brain damage — she was Cheyne-Stoking and they were sitting and watching her go. I called to her. She started awake, wide-eyed, and stared at me.

"Go outside," she told her husband. "Go, go." And the same to her father in Chinese. She watched them leave before speaking again.

"I am tired," she said. "I want to go, David. Do you understand, I want to go?"

"To go, Cha Nan?"

"I am tired, so tired. Can you let me go?"

She was flushed, sweaty, in the close-aired room, with me and the newspapers and the IV bottles, and the heavy presence of death. It reminded me of nothing so much as a scene from a novel or play, something one cannot believe could ex-

ist outside of art — the certainty of her desire for death, her
impassioned clarity after days of somnolence and fever.

"All right, Cha Nan," I said. And her eyes closed.

At the nurses' station, I was writing an order to increase
her morphine to fifteen milligrams every two to three hours
when Larry came by. He read over my shoulder.

"That isn't enough. Give her thirty."

I scratched out and rewrote.

He nudged me. "You're writing an order to kill that lady."

"I know."

"How's it feel?"

I looked at the order, in my crabbed handwriting. Larry
pushed up against me, his bulk close.

"Lousy," I said. "Cosign it."

"Give me your pen."

Later I came back into the room. It was the last day of my
subinternship, and I had been going around to my dozen patients, writing off-service notes and making sure all unfin-
ished business would be followed up. Again I had dictated the
letter for Cha Nan's father. I asked Maureen how Cha Nan
was.

"I gave her thirty of morphine. Her family's in there again.
She's talking with them."

"She's a brave lady," I said. "She knows, she really knows
it's all over." I entered the room. Small, dark people surrounded Cha Nan — her father, husband, three women I
hadn't seen before. And she was Cheyne-Stoking with such
shuddering finality that I was scared each breath would be
her last one.

I touched her arm; she jolted awake.

"Oh! I feel so good!" Eyes wide open, staring black and
unblinking, surveyed us.

"You were talking and fell asleep," said her husband.

"I thought . . . I thought I was dead," she said, in awe of us and herself. "I was dead — but look, I am not. I feel so good, so strong now. Oh, I'm so happy, I'm not dead."

I told her about the letter, which had assumed a peculiar importance to me, as if it were some sort of contract or waiver of responsibility; and it was a great relief to touch her hand, to hear, "Thank you, David."

Then she said, "I have to talk. Listen to what I have to say." And she spoke in Chinese to her family. I left her wide-eyed, unnaturally alert but opiated beyond pain. It was ten o'clock that Sunday night before I finished off-service notes and headed home.

The next morning, beginning my Hematology rotation, I was assigned two of my Oncology patients as consults — Dr. Odysseus, the Greek surgeon with lymphoma dying far from Athens, and Cha Nan. When I came by the nursing station to check her chart, one of the nurses, not Maureen, told me Cha Nan had just died.

"That's good," I said.

I went down the hall. Perhaps she had just died, victim to her third disease contracted in treatment of the second, contracted in treatment of the first, a Chad Godya of illness begun with "one kid, one kid" of Hodgkin's disease and culminating in a slow and agonized yielding to the Angel of Death (who had yet to yield to "the Holy One, blessed be He"). But already the low cart, disguised to look like a linen hamper, and the pointy-faced husband and shriveled father, and the three dark, short women had gone. I headed toward the room of Dr. Odysseus, still living, still dying.

Fire in the Hills

Ambrose was ready to kill us. Ambrose was nineteen and two hundred pounds and six foot three, and two hundred and eighty-four days of his life had been spent rotting in the Farm, a prison for the criminally insane. Now he was back in. Over the weekend he had been transferred from the county jail to the locked psychiatric ward at the county hospital where I was working as a medical student.

Even mad, Ambrose was beautiful. His coal black, smooth skin seemed African, not American, his forehead was broad, his arms massively muscled. He wore one of the orange jump-suits issued at the county jail, with grease and dirt rubbed in as deep as original sin. Ambrose's gaze turned from me to Dr. Walsh, my supervisor, then fixed before the door. Something we could not see fascinated him. From time to time he winced or laughed. The air stank. Both doors in the room were impossibly distant from me — one behind Ambrose, the other blocked by a metal desk. I tried to think of what to ask. My years of medical school anatomy and physiology and bio-chemistry were useless before the fear Ambrose put in me.

He jerked in the chair. I recoiled. Ambrose's neck was bruised purple where he had tried to strangle himself. First he had beaten another prisoner, then he choked himself with his big hands. That was when they brought him here.

"What . . . what happened, Ambrose?" I asked him.

He kept looking at the air before the door.

"At the jail. Why did they send you over here?"

Ambrose stared at Dr. Walsh. "He the doctor who sent me up to the Farm?"

"I don't think he's ever seen you before," I said.

"Bullshit," said Ambrose. He was eyeing Walsh from head to foot. "I remember that fucking spot on his face."

Dr. Walsh was sweating, but then, so was I. Red pepper-and-salt hair was brushed down over his forehead to his bushy eyebrows. On his temple was what Ambrose was talking about, a birthmark that was pink-red and raised, the size and shape of a jalapeño pepper. All the patients asked Walsh about it, and generally it didn't bother him. It matched Walsh's hair and complexion, making him look designer-coordinated, like the drapes and upholstery of some house on a dry California hillside. Usually Walsh was as blank as one of those California houses — imperturbable, motionless and opaque, revealing only surfaces set behind surfaces, one reflection moving behind another like the panes of glass in a sliding door. He was the kind of Californian Joan Didion writes about, a quiet and well-tanned and technical man; he drove a shiny BMW out of the foothills every morning up to the front of the Psychiatry building, where he would park in the ambulance-loading zone and enter morning rounds fifteen minutes late, with coffee cup and Marlboro Lights in hand, and he would sit down — quietly, calmly — to hear about the patients who had been admitted overnight. Nothing ruffled him.

But now Walsh looked as scared as I felt. It was obvious that Ambrose was working up to something, right before our eyes, and here we were, watching it build, awed by his beauty and the questions of when and to whom, and afraid to move. I was not surprised when Ambrose lunged forward at us, but I was surprised that his hands grabbed the chair as if it alone kept him from smashing our skulls. Veins snaked out over his forearms.

Voice shaking, Dr. Walsh said something.

"What?" said Ambrose.

Dr. Walsh said Ambrose was free to leave, that we didn't have any more questions for him.

"No questions for me?" Ambrose sank back in the chair. "I got questions for you. You going to send me to the Farm?"

"No," said Dr. Walsh.

"How do I know? Tell me how do I know."

Ambrose just stared. Nothing Walsh said could stop that murderous staring.

A minute later Ambrose broke loose from the chair, but his hands reached for the doorknob, not for our necks. He lumbered out of the room and stopped in the hall, confused. It was only after Walsh rushed to the door and locked it, and sank into Ambrose's chair, rolling his head back, that he said anything.

"Jesus," he said. The entire ruddy terrain of his face was drenched in sweat.

Then we heard screaming out in the hall.

Five psych techs, four holding one limb each, another on his head, were sitting on Ambrose by the time we got out to the nurses' station. In a moment or two they picked him up face down and ran him down the hall toward the seclusion room like a human battering ram. Someone went after them with the four-points, leather manacles with leather straps, which could be attached to the four corners of the mattress frame.

Guardino, a patient, was over by the nurses' station, holding his face. A scrawny Sicilian, Guardino was in for setting grass fires in the hills. He told us he burned churches, too.

I came up to him.

"Ambrose hit him," said Donna, the social worker. "See if he's all right."

He was holding his face, but he didn't even have a bloody nose when I pried his hands away.

Ambrose started screaming in the seclusion room.

"Ten of Haldol i.m.," said Dr. Walsh.

"Vitamin H," said Donna, smiling at me. Her boyfriend was a rock musician who once played for Jefferson Airplane, and she liked drugs. She was blond and wore an embroidered peasant blouse and no bra and a long skirt and leather sandals and her toenails were painted silver. "He'll shut up pretty soon."

That afternoon, when I was about to leave, I walked past the open door of the seclusion room. A nurse crouched by Ambrose's side, about to shoot him with more Haldol.

"You!" he called. I stopped in the doorway. He called me closer, and I came to stand above him. He strained against the leather straps, toward me, and I would remember for a long time the sound of his pleading. "Why don't you let my arm go? Come on, let my arm go. I want to scratch my face."

"I can't," I said.

"What's the matter? You afraid I'll punch you out? You afraid I'll kick you?"

I didn't say anything. I was feeling sick, sick in the stomach and sick of the whole place, and I didn't want anything more than to drive up the peninsula to the university and dive into the fifty-meter outdoor swimming pool where I swam a mile every afternoon and, as a summer project, was perfecting my flip turn.

"Let go my fucking hand!" He came at me, twisting, convulsing, with such a force of effort that he nearly flipped the whole bed on top of himself. He roared. First it was about his hand, then it was unintelligible. Then he started wailing his guts out. "I'll kill you! I mean *you,* motherfucker, *you!* When I get loose I'll kill you!"

I still worry over that day I sat with Dr. Walsh in a small green room in a county hospital in California, watching Ambrose and waiting for him to come at us, and I still don't know what to make of it. Something besides terror was present in that room, something that fascinated me in a way it is hard to sympathize with these days, now that I have a better idea of what psychosis is about and what cannot be done about it, and what the so-called antipsychotic medications are all about. But at that time the locked ward of that county hospital, ugly and stale-aired, in violation of fire codes and incidentally of human decency, seemed to tell of the failure of California. It fascinated me that the madness of the patients was so typically Californian. Every morning two or three new patients, overwhelmed by biology or life, came in. They had been picked up walking naked down a freeway and swinging a golf club, or for screaming nonstop in a home computer store, or for overdosing on angel dust. Some had committed spectacular, grisly crimes. Their lives were *National Enquirer* headlines:

WOMAN RUNS DOWN MAILMAN WITH SPORTSCAR
MOTHER AND GRANDMOTHER KICKED TO DEATH BY SON
BOARDS AIRPLANE WITHOUT TICKET, ASSAULTS STEWARDESS
HILLSIDE ARSONIST CONFESSES
ROCK-THROWING YOUTH SENT TO MENTAL WARD
PROF'S WIFE SLASHES WRISTS

Talking with them made one feel disturbed and befuddled, the way one feels after reading a Joan Didion essay — led toward one destination only to have the ground shift beneath you so you end up somewhere unexpected, full of anxiety. The pure products of America brought to the locked ward, crazy from PCP or schizophrenia, would stay only three or four days. On the ward they would sulk or cry or sleep or act according to the dictates of their madness, posturing like practitioners of T'ai Chi, speaking secret languages, leaving incomprehensible messages on pieces of paper. They would be shot with phenothiazines. Then they would be sent out to a halfway house with an acronym for a name or home or to jail or, depending on the vagaries of Medi-Cal and Social Security, be let loose to wander back on the streets from which they had come. The ones who didn't take their medications would come right back. The ones who spoke to God would continue speaking to God. Some bounced back to the ward every other week.

It was an odd place. Oddest of all was the attraction I felt toward it, this place where you could watch unraveled minds begin to come together again, which set you thinking about the brain, that strange organ in its bony box which somehow took dopamine and norepinephrine and serotonin and a dozen other mere chemicals and turned them into *thoughts*. The great bafflement here was not the existence of madness, but of sanity, of order, of reason. Why weren't we all mad? Somehow the idea got fixed in my head that I wanted to be a psychiatrist. The idea was so strong that through the rest of medical school, a dozen more rotations in Medicine and Surgery and Pediatrics, I couldn't get rid of it. All the rest, however interesting, would seem a diversion.

The next morning I was surprised to see Ambrose sitting at the table by the nurses' station, rolling cigarettes. The major therapeutic activity on the ward, if an unofficial one, involved the rolling of cigarettes. For some reason no one understood, the bureaucracy of the California mental health system was able to afford cans of tobacco and sheaves of rolling paper but not whole cigarettes, so patients who were not too psychotic spent much of their days rolling cigarettes on a little machine made of a metal frame and two dowels with a loop of canvas around them. A pack of papers and an open can of tobacco would sit on one side, a few cigarettes on the other; the completed product would soon disappear, distributed among patients. Since patients were not allowed to have matches, they would light each cigarette off the dying butt of the last.

Ambrose was doing a pretty good job with the little machine, despite his big, clumsy hands, and a pile of cigarettes sat off to one side. I kept my distance.

He even came to the group meeting we had every morning after rounds, carrying a tan and black can of Laredo tobacco and a packet of Zig-Zag rolling papers. He was grinning like a kid. During group he rolled himself half a dozen more cigarettes, fat in the middle and with tufts of tobacco sprouting from their ends. He interrupted Donna.

"Hey, anyone got a light?"

"Ambrose, please be quiet," said Donna. Someone handed him a cigarette so he could light up. A new patient, a young Arab, was talking about why he had ended up in the hospital. The night before, after holding his wife hostage for five hours, he had surrendered to police and was brought in. There was no gun; they found him in a closet. All this had made the papers and the evening news. Now he wanted to apologize to his wife, but she was gone, spending the day in Marine World with her brother, forgetting.

"Why is he here? He's here because he's crazy like the rest of us," said Ambrose. "Can I talk?"

"Let Mohammed talk first."

Mohammed started crying.

Ambrose stood up and walked to the door. He took the cigarette he was smoking and lit another one in his hand. He made a move to offer it to someone, but no one would take it, so he just stood with two cigarettes burning in his hands.

"When you-all going to let me out of here?"

"Ambrose, you're interrupting."

He looked sharply at me, all boyishness leaving his face. "Look, man, I been in the hospital two hundred and eighty-five days. And I want to get out of here. You understand?"

"This is group meeting," I said. "You want to stay or go?"

He looked at the cigarette in his hand. "I want to think about it for a while."

The next day in group meeting he had some suggestions for another patient, an unkempt, sallow kid who kept telling us he didn't care what happened to him.

"What do you mean?" Ambrose said. "Ain't you got a check coming? Or ain't you even together enough to sign up for your money? You know what, man, I tell you what you should do. Number one, wash your greasy hair. Number two, shave them whiskers off. You ain't got enough hair to grow a beard. Number three . . . number three, take a shower. Number four —"

"You really have it all worked out for him, Ambrose," I said.

Ambrose grinned; everyone laughed.

By this time we had gotten to like Ambrose. The Haldol or something had knocked the anger back for a while, and he was so charming and beautiful that everyone liked him. That day, we had a barbecue, prepared by the patients, for both patients and staff. The tossed salad had cinders in it, the carrots-and-raisins-with-mayonnaise tasted soapy, and the hamburgers had been patted into odd shapes by hands I preferred not to think about, but we all went into the courtyard for lunch — Dr. Walsh and Donna and the psych techs and I. Guardino bounced a worn basketball off his hairy knees, alternating left and right and shouting to God in Italian. A new patient, a black-haired woman in a loose bathrobe, was screaming at full pitch. *"Animal. Stop. House. Left turn. Saturday. One step. Andrea. Crystal. K-k-k-k-k-krystal. Stop!"* But no one paid any attention to her. Donna had twisted her ankle, and she sat soaking her bare foot in a bedpan of hot water. I came by, carrying a soggy paper plate of food and saw Ambrose by her side, holding her hand. She let him, even though by now we knew that what he was sent up to the Farm for was rape.

"I ain't going to hurt you or push you or scratch you or do nothing to you," he was saying to her. "That girl, she lied to me. I got sent away for something I didn't do, and I ain't touched ground since."

Dr. Walsh came up to me, and we started talking. We seemed closer after what happened with Ambrose. He said affably to me, loud enough that Ambrose could have heard it if he had not been watching Donna so closely, "It's hard to know what to do with someone like him."

The next day Ambrose's seventy-two hours were up and he wanted to leave. Charges from the county jail — whatever they were — had been dropped, and since he didn't look as though he was going to kill anyone immediately we had to let him go. The most we could offer him was a bus ticket to El Guyas, where his cousin, an ex-forward for the Lakers, lived, and where his father sometimes drifted through.

"Call El Guyas," Ambrose said. "So they can tell my dad to loaf around the bus station to pick me up when the bus gets in."

We talked about why he needed to take his medications even though they made him stiff.

"I want to be loose as a goose," said Ambrose. "I'm all tied up right now."

"Look, man," said Donna, "we understand. But you've got to take your meds or you'll be right back in here."

"I know that," Ambrose said. "You think you could give me a ride to the bus station?"

"We can call you a cab."

"No thanks," said Ambrose. "I'll walk."

"It's a long way. It's a hell of a long way."

"I just want to walk and think in the blue sky. I got plenty of time. I just got to take care of business."

"We can only give you ten days worth of medications," I said. "You'll have to get a refill down in El Guyas."

"I know that," he said. "But first I'm going to see what's happening here in the valley. I got a lot of friends here, thirty or forty at least." When he started talking, Ambrose had been all lit up, grinning; now he was solemn enough to punch me.

Finally, he shuffled out of the office. He stopped a moment, staring at whatever it was we could not see, then walked away.

"He won't take them," I said.

"He might," Donna said.

"He's got a lousy prognosis," said Dr. Walsh.

Later, during coffee break, I looked out the window and saw Ambrose, a distant, dark figure, slowly walking around the dry shrubbery, way over by the Crisis Center. Walsh and I were talking differential diagnosis on the new, screaming woman, and we talked for half an hour before Ambrose disappeared.

The next morning Donna limped into the office looking upset.

"Did he finally go?" she said. "When I left last night he was out there in the parking lot, by my car. You know, he stalks women, that's why he was in jail. I hope he doesn't know where I live. How do you think he knew which car was mine?"

For the next few days I checked around my car, as well, before getting in; I recalled what Ambrose said he'd do when he was mad, and he might, too. But we never saw him again.

Children of the Valley

I . FEBRUARY

RAIN. Rain falls over the flat expanses of the valley, over the
small trees and the monotonous low houses, effaces the rolling hills across the bay we cannot see. February rain. It comes
down for hours, late in arriving but persistent as disease. We
are in the fourth-floor ICU, the Pediatric Intensive Care Unit,
crowded around the bed of a splotchy baby.

"I don't understand it," says Izzy, our resident, who wears
a Spiderman pin in the lapel of his white coat. He is gloomy
and pale, with limp brown hair falling over his eyes and a
thick mustache that hides most of his mouth. "He's not tach-
ing with the Levophed anymore." He turns to the nurse. "Is
his MAP standardized yet?"

His pressure is twenty; eighty is survival.

"It's standardized," the nurse says.

"Zero it again," Izzy tells her.

"What difference is a millimeter or two going to make?"

He shrugs. "Mike," he asks the intern, "did you call the
parents yet?"

"I talked to the mother. She's coming."

"What about the father?"

"He's a basket case, he's not going to come in. She'll want to see the baby alone for a while."

"Fine," Izzy says.

A blood gas comes back: pH 7.00, pCO_2 77, pO_2 31, bicarb 11. I read it off and everyone becomes silent.

"Thirty-one?"

I nod. "How about some more bicarb?"

Izzy glares at me. He rolls his mustache in his lower teeth. It's my second day on the service, and up to now he hasn't really noticed me.

"Sure, do it. What the hell. Nothing else is doing any good."

When they give the bicarb nothing happens. Robby, the baby, is a two-year-old who had a bad cough that turned into pneumonia that turned into generalized sepsis, poisoning his entire body. He lies on his back, spread-limbed, with tubes and lines entering his body. His skin is marbled with blue. On the view boxes, X rays show his whited-out lungs. It's a wonder that the respirator is able to pump even 31 millequivalents of oxygen into his blood.

Beside Robby is another baby, Alyssa Montero, who drowned when her mother left her in the bath to answer the phone; when she returned Alyssa was floating facedown, dead. But she brought Alyssa to the hospital anyway, someone pumped the water out of her lungs, and fifteen minutes later she was alive, defying scientific fact. Now she lies in a crib with white metal bars, gurgling at the mobile above her. She has shaggy dark hair and large, intelligent black eyes, and she laughs now as I tickle her, moving arms and legs easily; as we've put in the chart, there are "no focal neurological signs." I wiggle the mobile, and she follows the little plastic ducks and rabbits with her hands. A commotion causes me to turn.

Robby has arrested. On the monitor his heart rate is 28 and irregular, his MAP is 14, and the nurse is attempting CPR by pushing on his chest while Izzy injects drugs through the central line.

"Do we have epi in an intracardiac syringe?" he asks. "Where's the mother? Is the mother here yet?" His eyes fix on me, standing useless, awed. "Find the mother."

In the waiting room are two Mexican women, both young, fat or pregnant, or both. I ask if they've seen the mother; they tell me in Spanish that they do not know English. I ask the nurses at the front desk; they haven't seen her. I call the operator and have her paged *stat*. Then I stand by the door of the ICU, ready to intercept her and direct her. I wait five minutes by my digital watch, as the two women gossip in Spanish. Then I go inside.

Izzy is by the nurses' station.

"I couldn't . . ." I say.

He shrugs and turns back to the phone.

The code is over. The nurses are back at the other cribs, the students are in a side room, and a white screen has been pulled around Robby's bed. I walk around it. All the tubes have been detached, and the baby has been wrapped in a white blanket, so only the face and one mottled hand stick out. The only other dead baby I ever saw was in anatomy class, a pretty blond girl with no visible reason for not being alive.

The two Mexican ladies come in. They bump against me and crowd their fat bellies against Alyssa's crib, and without a glance at the white screen begin cooing and calling to Alyssa. In this light, a weird product of fluorescent tubing and gray rain, I see they are not identical after all, but that one is slovenly and middle-aged and the other is young — perhaps nineteen — and pretty and pregnant. I wonder which of them is the mother.

We are at a public hospital in a California valley, a hospital for the poor. There are hills on three sides of us, a bay somewhere to the north, and the ground is flat, like the bottom of a lake risen above water after many millennia, land that is solid but somehow still aquatic. The freeways are elevated here — perhaps the water is expected to rise again. The air, when it does not rain, smells of onions or maybe it is garlic; Izzy says there is a factory south of us, somewhere in the hills.

Thursday, after rounds, we come into the playroom for a teaching session. Students and house officers, we sit in chairs designed for toddlers. Knees crowd up against our faces, our white coats fan out on the floor. From the hall we can hear the faint, muffled sounds of crying babies and beeping monitors and the ringing of telephones and the voices of harried nurses. I think of Robby.

"Dr. O'Halloran's going to talk fluids," says Mike, who sits in a tiny plastic chair. "Prepare to be confused."

Izzy comes inside; his white coat and hair are drenched. He sits down on a wooden rocking horse and rests his chin on its head.

"What's with you?" Mike says.

"I was out at my car," Izzy says.

"Again?" says Mike. "Jesus Christ!"

Izzy rocks back and forth on the horse, disconsolate.

"He died with bad lytes," Mike says. "Sodium 120, potassium 7.5. We really screwed up giving him the extra K."

"And the quarter normal saline," Izzy says.

"Don't blame yourselves," says Emily, our senior resident. She is an elegant, remote woman, a Bostonian who seems entirely out of place in the valley.

"Oh, I don't," says Izzy. "The kid was dead when he hit the ER. Still . . ." He rocks back and forth. "That reminds me of a joke. A great Yiddish joke. You want to hear it?" No one says anything, so he goes on. "You see, an old tailor is walking down the street and finds a bag containing a hundred thousand dollars. He can't believe it! He takes the money home and wraps it in a blanket and stuffs it behind his refrigerator . . ."

It is a long joke, about a gun and a rabbi and a thief, and it is several minutes before he reaches the punch line: "The rabbi tells him, 'He says you can go to the devil.' "

Nobody laughs but me. To me it seems wonderful, justifying, or at least excusing, the morning.

"That's horrible," Emily says.

Izzy rocks on the horse, now in a foul mood.

"Shit!" he says. "Why didn't they send him somewhere else? Why'd he have to die on my hands?"

No one says anything.

"Where the hell's O'Halloran?" Izzy asks.

After lunch we go down to Pathology. Lunch was linguica, long gristly Portuguese sausages, and my stomach rumbles as I follow Izzy and Mike downstairs to the basement — Pathology departments always seem to be underground — past the clanging pipes of the furnace room, through a door marked No Admittance.

It is an immense relief to find only a few organs on the steel table: lungs, liver, a heart. Small, child-sized organs. A pale woman in a plastic smock — a Pathology resident — shows us the fatal hemorrhage in the lungs. It is anticlimactic. It turns out Mike and the pale woman went to medical school together in LA; and they trade stories about who dropped out to have babies, who's becoming a hotshot academician, which couples have been made and unmade.

Izzy and I leave Mike there talking.

"What do you think?" Izzy says when we're at the furnace room again.

"I've seen it before," I say.

"That reminds me," Izzy says. "When I was in med school. We had these patients come in, Arabs, a whole damn family all with the same name." I wonder what on earth reminded him of this, or for that matter what reminded him of the rabbi story, but think better of asking.

"They were all named Ibrahim and Muhammed, with four names. Ibrahim Muhammed Muhammed Ibrahim — Ibrahim was their last name — and Muhammed Ibrahim Muhammed Ibrahim, and Muhammed Muhammed Muhammed Ibrahim. It was incredible. Calling the lab was a nightmare. Bed Control went crazy. Muhammed Muhammed Muhammed — Hey, that reminds me. . . ."

The children here are small, they have no history, they can be examined in two minutes. They are delicate, though, and it takes much practice to thread plastic tubes into their thin-walled little veins. But I don't have to do much of that. Worst is that they are victims, so many of them, abused, mistreated, cruelly malformed. One does one's best to comfort them, to approach them calmly and with love, if one can comfort one's own fears.

It is unsettling to hear them cry. They are always screaming and crying, but hoarsely, automatically, without much hope. You cannot save them all.

II. MARCH

Outside, the freeways roar, the hills are lost in haze. Inside, the babies in their mist tents have disappeared in white fog, so that only occasionally does a pale hand appear through the mist, clutching at the plastic wall. A paralyzed girl roars down the hall in her motorized wheelchair, guided by a rubber disc held in her mouth.

"I can't believe it," I say. I show Izzy the chart I've been reading. "Fifteen years old — it says she weighs twenty-seven pounds."

"They must mean kilos," Izzy says.

"No, it says pounds. Underlined."

We look at each other and laugh. My white coat sticks to my back, my hair against my forehead. It's just like summer in the Midwest, an inversion of sky so that clouds rest on the ground, which is hot as though the sun is blazing underneath.

"She must be a midget," I say.

"Mike's gone to pick her up," Izzy says. "Transport from Saint Barrabas."

The girl in the wheelchair, who has a moon face with bulging cheeks and a bridgeless nose, stops for a moment by us, then roars down the straightaway.

"C-three section," Izzy says.

"What?"

"Her spinal cord, severed at C-three, up in the neck. No one knows how she breathes."

"Jesus," I say. An image arises in my mind, from Fellini's *Satyricon* — two dwarfs, both double amputees, the legless man riding on the armless man's shoulders, held by a leather harness. A rude Italian joke. It's as though I haven't really *seen* the sick kids before today, not the really sick ones who won't ever become whole, the ones who make Pediatrics so much sadder than Medicine.

"Here's Mike," says Izzy. The wheelchair girl maneuvers to let them pass: Mike and a white-suited ambulance driver pushing a gurney with our twenty-seven-pound patient. They turn at the desk and pass toward the ICU. All I see of the patient is a head. The rest, what there is, is covered with a bulky red blanket.

We follow them inside.

To transfer her to the bed they have stripped off the blanket. She is not a midget.

"Oh. My. God." Izzy says three sentences. She is naked.

"Not so loud."

Izzy gestures to me to get the IV bottle. The plastic tubing moves across this Giacometti figure, this abstraction of the human form, this giant fetus, pink skeleton. I hesitate to describe her more. I am not shy about looking, though, as I hold the IV bottle above my head: she is alive, she *moves* on the bed.

"Let's get the fluids running," says Izzy. "Come on, man. Turn it on. A hundred cc's an hour. Let it all drip in."

I open it up all the way.

In truth, I don't recall Robby's death anymore; I've seen enough others that it's been erased. But it is here in my notes, so it must have happened.

I don't know about the twenty-seven-pounder, either, whether she survived.

"Where is Dr. Chalupa?" asks the interpreter, a short woman in blue polyester. "The parents say Dr. Chalupa was going to take care of their baby."

The parents stand beside the baby's crib. The mother, a careworn middle-aged woman, looks at me with a kind of patient loathing; and the father, mustached, stout, in an old windbreaker, stares at the floor. Neither of them speaks English.

"Tell them," I say, "that Dr. Chalupa may come and visit, but that the house staff will be taking care of the baby." No one here has heard of Dr. Chalupa.

The interpreter explains in Spanish, and the parents respond with passion and anger. She says, "They have been here before and they have had a very bad experience. They feel that the doctors were experimenting on their baby."

"Experimenting?" I say. For the first time I get a good look at the baby propped in its crib. It is not a baby but rather a small monster, with low ears, a flat, bridgeless nose, a hairline scarcely an inch above its close-set eyes. It makes a repetitive cry that might be that of a normal baby if it were not so divorced from anguish. And it rocks, back and forth, with motions of its stunted, muscular limbs. "Can you explain," I say, "that we want to take care of the baby. We're not going to experiment."

"They do not want any tests done."

"I'm sure we'll have to do some. Blood tests, a chest X ray."

She does not even have to consult this time; the mother shakes her head no.

I sigh. "Tell her to wait. I'll go get my resident."

I can't find Izzy, but Emily, the senior resident, is at the nurses' station. I explain the situation, watching her delicately immobile face. She has auburn hair, and a smooth face covered entirely with freckles a shade lighter than her hair, and an expression of complete, unperturbable self-possession, grounded in generations, so I have heard, of Back Bay sovereignty. She comes from the Mayflower on both sides. She never plays with the babies.

"Why is the child here?" she asks.

"Possible pneumonia, versus congestive heart failure."

"Let me go talk to them."

When we return to the room the parents are standing at the crib, trying to quiet the baby.

"They are going to take the baby home," says the interpreter.

Emily begins speaking to the parents — in Spanish. The

parents cannot be as surprised as I am to hear her, fluent, controlled, soothing. I wonder where on earth she learned this. She bargains with the mother. They are two women in a market haggling over a fish or an embroidered shirt, the mother passionate and outraged, Emily deft and cool. Finally she turns to me.

"I think we've got it. We'll admit the baby but we won't do any tests without consulting them and explaining everything. All right?"

"Sure."

Watched by the suspicious parents, I examine the baby. It cries as I touch it, pushing me away with dwarfish thick hands, grunting, moaning, sniffling through its snotty nose — a hairless rodent trapped in a human body. I know the parents' anger must grow from love, but when I think of this creature and the twenty-seven-pounder and the nine-month-old baby who has never left the Intensive Care Unit since birth, who has been fed through a hole in his belly so long he has forgotten how to suck — it seems it would be a mercy to . . . to what? Drown them like cats in a burlap sack, thrown off a bridge? I shake those thoughts away. Ridiculous. We're here to help.

I examine, I touch, I fight the grasping clutch of the baby, Teresa. I shine a light in its eyes and it shakes its head like a dog. The parents step close. I finish in a rush.

At the nurses' station I find Emily resting against the counter. She looks up without curiosity as I approach.

"I learned Spanish in Seville," she says. "I find it useful here in the valley."

In the morning a professor from the main hospital, Dr. de Vita, arrives. He is a wiry, excitable Italian. I present a patient with nephrotic syndrome, whom we discuss for a few minutes; then he interrupts me.

"I am sorry, I have nothing to add," he says. "This sort of

patient I am not interested in. Have you any congenital anomalies instead?"

I look at Emily. "Teresa. She's a funny-looking baby."

"Funny? How is funny?" De Vita rises from his chair, agitated, with what might seem to be fury but is, I see, feverish interest.

"Well, she's a two-and-a-half-year-old child, who presents with possible pneumonia —"

"I am not interested. I want to know, what are her findings? How far apart are her eyes? What is her skull circumference? Is her upper trunk large or small compared to her legs? How are her ears shaped? Well?"

Everyone turns to me.

"I didn't measure head circumference."

"My God! You didn't measure? You can tell me nothing. Come, I only have a few minutes, let's see the baby. Do you have a tape measure?"

Tense and passionate, he herds us into Teresa's room, grabs a paper tape measure.

"Amazing!" he says. "Look at this — epicanthic folds, low-set ears, decreased skull circumference. And see, the skin . . ." He pinches her belly, her ribs. "It has the loose elasticity of the Ehlers-Danlos syndrome, but it is not typical of Ehlers-Danlos — the joints are hyperflexible, yet . . . yet . . ."

I burn in embarrassment. Emily, across the crib, looks at me blandly. I want to despise her but am incapable of anything except awe and yearning.

"Tell me," says de Vita, "what studies are you doing on this baby?"

"Well, the parents don't want her to be —"

"I don't care. What are the results?"

Surprisingly, Emily talks. "It *is* a very touchy situation with the family."

"How is ignorance better than knowledge?" asks de Vita.

"What good will it do the family to know?" Emily says. "There's no cure for what she has."

De Vita glares at us. "I am late for a meeting. I have to leave. But this child, she is fascinating, she is wonderful. Do studies. Chromosome analysis, urine-reducing substances, fibroblast cultures. And measure everything. See why she is so small. When did she stop growing? This is fascinating. What again is the baby's name?"

"Teresa."

That evening, after dinner, the father comes by. I explain through the interpreter that the baby has neither heart failure nor pneumonia, only a bad cough. The father seems disappointed. He tells the interpreter he is tired of the experiments and is taking Teresa home. Izzy and even Emily cannot stop him.

The next morning, after rounds, I am paged to the nurses' station. The clerk is placating someone over the phone when I get there.

"You called me?"

"Yes. It is a Dr. Chalupa. He is calling about Teresa."

"She went home."

"She went home," the clerk says. "Yes, if you would like to talk to someone the medical student is here." She looks at me. "I see. All right. Thank you. Goodbye." She hangs up. "A Dr. Chalupa. He did not want to talk to a medical student."

Midnight of my night on, I lie down for a while in the "submarine" — a small, windowless room between the Pediatric Nursery and the Obstetrics ward, with lockers on one side, a bed on the other, a bathroom at one end. The walls reverberate, and I hear echoes of every breath I take, and a watch inside one of the lockers is as loud as a kitchen timer. From somewhere very close I hear a woman in labor. "Oh my God, oh my God, oh my God!" Lying curled, with my head toward the wall, I imagine her on the other side of the wall, flat on her back, big bellied, fecund, sweating. She cries, and I lie in my sweaty greens, trying to sleep. Then I hear, "Pediatrician to Delivery *stat!*"

I make myself get up, put on shoes and glasses, stumble out to the ward.

"Action's over in OB," says a voice behind me.

The night clerk. A girl with a schoolbook. I run past her to OB.

Izzy is waiting with a towel in his hands. The obstetrician is hard at work.

"Just in time," he says. "This is a heavy mec stainer, a thirty-two-weeker with PROM, mother febrile to 102 degrees, and they're having a hell of a time getting the kid out." Mec, which clogs lungs, is meconium, feces, expelled in distress before birth.

I hear "Oh God! Oh my God!" and "Push! Push!"

It doesn't come out well. It doesn't pink up like the ones I've seen before; in fact it hardly moves when Izzy rams the ET tube down its throat.

"Suck!" he calls. "Come on, damn it, suck!" The nurse joggles the baby's plum-colored limbs, which move feebly. "Bag it, bag it, then suction. Let's get this mec *out*." She squeezes the mask to the baby's face, pumps hard.

He sees me on the periphery.

"Go on over to the nursery; tell them we've got a heavy mec stainer coming."

When I return, he says, "What do you think its Apgars were?"

"Five and six?"

He shakes his head. "Two and five. This kid stinks. The

mom weighs two hundred and twenty pounds; didn't even know she was pregnant. Doesn't want to see the kid."

I see her in the room, mountainous and immobile. The tiny Indian Obstetrics resident, with red forehead dot showing below her blue cap, still works between her legs. The mother's head is turned away from us, toward the wall.

"Okay, let's bag this kid on the way over to the nursery," Izzy says.

I follow.

III. APRIL

I have been rotated to the Outpatient clinics, where I spend mornings in a small office on a long, sunny corridor, seeing babies with coughs and earaches, using my few words of Spanish to ask about formulas and immunizations. This is a happier place. Fifteen-year-olds play with their babies, crackling gum. Grandmothers gossip. I ask those who know enough English about car seats. Do they know how many babies fly loose in cars, hitting their heads, breaking their small bodies? They should be strapped in for sudden stops. I hand out pamphlets about car seats. Nights I'm on call in the Emergency Room.

One night I'm on call with Izzy. I haven't seen Izzy much this month, except occasionally in the cafeteria or a conference, or, more often, out the window of my examining room, from a distance, on his way out to the parking lot, or coming back in. Some days he goes back and forth several times. I'm struck tonight by how lousy Izzy looks, pale, gray-skinned, tired, and I wonder if I look the same. I do have a persistent scratching at the back of my throat — probably some virus picked up from the kids — and I'm tired most of the time.

Tonight we see a Samoan baby with a cold, and a little black girl born without arms. We give the little armless girl's mother a prescription for Ampicillin, then sit in the glass-enclosed nurses' cubicle, eating dinner on trays from the cafeteria.

Izzy tells me about North Dakota, where he'd been before he came here.

"It was intense," he says. "Seven of us running a fifty-bed hospital in the middle of nowhere. We were together twenty-four hours a day, so any little thing could build up until someone was annihilated. I saw it happen. You made a little mistake and somebody would get on your back. I saw a guy, a really smart guy, a good doc, get torn apart by another guy who just had a grudge. It was a little different for me, of course, because I had a wife and kid."

"Had?" I say.

"Well, she's in Dakota still."

I consider asking him about the kid, and decide not to.

"She came out here for a while," he says. "Four months into my internship. She left in a week."

"Oh," I say. "You going back to North Dakota when you finish?"

"I'm not going to finish," he says. "At least not next year. I need to make some money, and spend some time with my kid."

"Sounds like a good life," I say.

He looks at me strangely, and something seems to break free in him.

"My time's not my own," he says. "My wife and I are divorcing, and I have the kid right now. He's three. I've got to be a better mother for him than his mother can be. I mean, what judge would say to a mother who wants a kid, who's willing to spend all day at home with him, that she can't have him?"

"That's terrible," I say. "That's a terrible situation. You really want your kid, huh."

He's almost crying. I'm embarrassed. I look down at the cornhusks piled to the side of my plate, and the sludge of refried beans.

"Listen," he says. "Why don't you go back to the Peds section, see if there's any more patients. I've got to go out to my car."

"Again?" I say, but he's gotten up already, leaving his tray behind.

In cubicle 12 there's a three-year-old girl with an earache. Her left tympanic membrane bulges. Simple: Ampicillin for ten days. I examine, diagnose, reassure, then go out in search of Izzy. I find Izzy in cubicle 1, right in front of the nurses' station, where the sickest cases go; he's staring at a man lying in bed. He is a middle-aged man with black hair, and his skin is blanched, and his bare feet look like porcelain, and his chest runs with sweat.

"See?" Izzy whispers. "This is Dr. Xavier, one of our attendings."

"You're kidding."

"No. Came in with nausea and vomiting, severe chest pain. After work. Just closed up his office . . . His nurse found him sitting in his car. He's fifty-four years old."

The ER resident comes up with the EKG. It shows an acute myocardial infarction, multiple PVCs, complete left bundle branch block.

"Jesus," says Izzy. "He's a pediatrician. A really dedicated guy; works with poor families in the barrio. This isn't supposed to happen to pediatricians," he says. "Shit! A surgeon has a heart attack, you expect it — he killed himself. But the family doc in the valley . . ."

"Didn't smoke or drink," says the ER resident. "He's in good shape, too."

The Medicine resident comes down, and the Surgery resident after him. Dr. Xavier lies motionless on the gurney, the nurse trying to get another IV into his waxy right hand.

"Forget it. We'll do it in the OR. Let's go. We're going to get a balloon in him."

"He's going to die," Izzy says.

Soon they wheel Dr. Xavier away. I'm shaken myself. It's altogether too much, another story starting when you're least ready for it, unavoidable, a lesson in mortality that is altogether redundant.

A diabetic girl comes in just as the earache leaves. Fortunately she keeps us busy until midnight. Then there's nothing.

"This your last night?" Izzy asks.

I tell him yes. I get my coat and backpack.

"Well, I wanted to tell you, you did a really good job here. Hey, you going out now?"

I nod.

"Let me walk with you," he says.

"Sure."

We walk out of the ER. Izzy tests his beeper.

"I've got to go to my car," he says.

"Again? How come you're always going to your car?"

"Oh, I keep my dog there," Izzy explains.

I don't believe him.

"Yeah, I do," he says. "I had another dog which I kept at home but he got stolen. So I keep this one in my car. I park in the shade. He's a crazy dog. After the first couple days, he *wanted* to be in the car. Now he can hardly stand it out of the car. He's a really crazy dog."

I shake my head. We're past the waiting room now and outside, in the humid valley air. There's a vague pain in my chest, or more in my upper midbelly, as though someone had elbowed me there. Most likely it's from the refried beans and enchiladas, but it's bad enough to make me hunch over as we walk.

"I come out and feed him and take him for walks any chance

I get," Izzy says. I head off toward my car, he turns toward his. "Hey, you did a good job, a really good job," he calls after me. "I mean it."

"He made it onto the balloon all right," says Cindy, who is in my class in med school. She'd been doing Cardiology at the valley when I was on Peds. We're back up at the university now, away from the scorched valley — in fact, we're sitting on the edge of the grassy bank beside the outdoor swimming pool, watching people do their laps. It's warm now; just in the last few days has it been pleasant enough to sit and sun, and there are families at the far end of the pool, mothers and babies and toddlers on blankets. Suburban families. And in the water, three little boys splashing one other and a father holding a little girl, teaching her to float. She splashes and giggles and squeals.

"His MAP was only fifty and his wedge was something incredible — thirty-eight, forty — but he was perfusing all right. But around three A.M. he just arrested and that was it. It's too bad. He really hadn't been having chest pain or anything," Cindy says. "Just dull pressure that came and went. Not even angina. He was thinking of going to his doctor the next week to have it checked out. There wasn't much reason to worry."

I lie back and look at the sun. Hard to believe it's the same star that shines down on the valley.

Touching

"SCOOT DOWN to the edge of the table, hon," says Dr. Snarr. The small room is hot, the air stuffy. Our patient winces at the word *hon*. She is a young woman with chronic pelvic pain, the bane of gynecologists, and I can tell she doesn't like Snarr's tone. She does scoot along the table, though, and Snarr kicks a wheeled stool toward me. I sit on it, slide between her legs, ready for my lesson of the day. Feet and calves and thighs surround me, suddenly very close. Snarr positions the lamp before my chest, so light pours on her. I warm the speculum in my gloved hand and, with a twist, insert it.

"Open it up," he says. "Tighten it all the way open. Pull down to keep away from the urethra. You hit the urethra and no patient will ever come back to you."

Snarr is my teacher, a gaunt and narrow-shouldered man with a small potbelly below the belt of his corduroy pants. Before coming in here, he went over the information I had gathered and insisted it was nonsense. She couldn't possibly feel that kind of pain. I must not be asking the right questions. Hadn't I learned anything? Gynecologists traditionally have the reputation of being the dummies of medicine: surgeons laugh at their clumsiness in the operating room, internists at their ignorance of medical fact, psychiatrists at their insensitivity. And so far Snarr had done nothing to dispel that prejudice, which was too bad, considering that I was an impressionable third-year medical student, still trying to decide what field to select.

"Okay," says Snarr. "Now swab it out real well. Get some cells on that."

I swab.

"Pull that speculum out now. Get a good look at those walls."

I see pink folds as I pull, pink, moist walls bulging against the metal of the speculum — aquatic territory, the scalloped forms of submarine life. It's out. Snarr is quick next with lubricating jelly on the first two fingers of my glove. I stand up, push the stool away. I begin the manual exam.

"*Aiee!*" The woman screams and slides up on the table. "God! Oh God!"

"So that's . . . that's where it hurts," I say. I'm sweating. "Just . . . just a second, I'll try more gently."

I feel around again. This time she doesn't scream. She breathes deeply. I can't feel a damn thing, but with Snarr watching I can't pull out right away. For a month I've been spending afternoons in the gynecology clinic with Dr. Snarr — a month of women's bottoms on the edges of tables, of the hot lamp in front of my chest, the examining glove on my hand, powdered inside, the smells of femaleness. And the confidences of women, fascinating and at times overpowering, about their pains, their periods, their fertility, their husbands, their lovers. What gets to me, though, are the exams. The touching. Deep internal touching, feeling for the bulge of the uterus, for those small elusive olives the ovaries, exploring for tenderness, creating sudden moments of pain. Technically I'm reasonably good, as good as can be expected for a third-year medical student rotating through Ob-Gyn. But I still find it strange to be touching intimately but without passion — as a doctor.

I'm not alone in this either; the other medical students on Ob-Gyn seem just as awkward as I. We hang around in the lounge, where the pharmaceutical rep sometimes leaves free coffee and doughnuts, cracking jokes, laughing too much.

It reminds me of another situation, in the second-year physical diagnosis course, where we had to examine each other. The new idea that year was that we'd learn how to be more compassionate doctors if we practiced physical exams on one another first, before going on to patients.

We were divided into small groups, men and women together, and sent to various examining rooms. Our exams began at the head and worked down. You couldn't get too upset about looking into your medical student buddy's eyes, but by the second session, when we got down to the chest, the protests began. First the women complained and refused to be examined, but as it became clear that genital and rectal exams were also part of the required curriculum, men started to protest as well. Finally there was a full-scale revolt. A petition was circulated, meetings were hurriedly arranged with various administrators, protests were loud and vocal. The class was boycotted. We ended up learning the pelvic exam on professional models and doing rectal exams on plastic dummies. No one felt the course should be repeated.

I've always been sort of puzzled why my fellow medical students got so upset. After all, we had done just about everything together — cut open cadavers, crammed for exams, played touch football on the front lawn, dated and flirted and confided and complained. What it comes down to, I think, was that after two years together in med school, we knew each other too well, far too well for touching to be neutral. To palpate, percuss, auscultate, and probe each other's bodies brought out too many undoctorly thoughts.

We were a long way, I realize now, from learning the doctor's dispassionate touch. But the real problem came when our teachers were no better than we — when they were clumsy and awkward, too.

"All right," Dr. Snarr says, "let me try my hand." He steps in. I strip off my glove and wash my hands, ready to observe a deft exam, pinpointing the source of pain, exploring yet reassuring.

But in a second the woman is screaming, writhing on the table. Snarr is reaching way far in, clumsily it seems, pushing so hard her hips rise from the table; and she is crying, grabbing the table with her hands. I feel sick just watching. I have no way of knowing what, if anything, Snarr is finding, since he does not explain.

"All right, hon," he tells her. He pulls off his glove. "Wipe yourself off; we'll come back and see you in a minute.

"I don't know why the heck she hurts," he says when we are outside. "Give her some estrogen cream."

She'd dressed when I come back in. She's pale and woozy, and there's still pain in her eyes. I hand her the prescription.

"Come back if it gets worse," I say.

"Than what?" the woman asks.

I am embarrassed. I murmur something, that I'm sorry we didn't come up with anything. Then I hurry out after my teacher.

I find him in the side room, having coffee and doughnuts, courtesy of the pharmaceutical rep. The next patient isn't ready yet.

"Have some," he says.

I decline. I'm too jittery to eat.

"That girl," says Dr. Snarr. "What do you think her problem is?"

I consider the possibilities: pelvic inflammatory disease, endometriosis, cysts. I talk, but I don't say what I really think: that he has no sense of what he put her through. That he's insensitive. Clumsy. A jerk. I'm disappointed, too, but I'm not sure why.

Perhaps it's that I wished he was a better doctor, a better role model. Certainly not all gynecologists are like Dr. Snarr, but at that moment it seemed as though they were. And what I needed so much was to know how to be with patients, how to deal with the feelings they evoked, how to make them feel at ease. If Dr. Snarr had been a better teacher, I might conceivably have gone into his field.

Dr. Snarr washes down the rest of his doughnut.

"So what else have we got out there?" he says.

A young black woman in a white gown looks around nervously as we enter.

"Scoot down to the edge of the table, hon," says Snarr.

Wincing at the word *hon,* the woman nevertheless scoots down.

Snarr kicks the wheeled stool over toward me.

And I begin.

Related Illnesses

"CALL six-six-two-five. Call six-six-two-five."

Internship. Every night on call it was the same thing. Down seventeen flights in the elevator to the basement, get dinner out of the machines, sit down to eat. And my beeper would go off. I'd never know what it might be — a heart stopped, a blood pressure falling. Anything. Or nothing. Either way, nerves jangled, anxiety rose. I left my soggy ham sandwich, my bitter Coke in a paper cup, and hurried to the telephone.

"What's up?" I said.

"You the intern up here tonight?" It was Ernie. Ernie was a senior resident in Medicine, working on another service. His grandmother, Mrs. Jonas, was a patient on our floor, and he was always flipping through her chart or examining her, always second-guessing us.

"Yeah, what is it?" I said, trying to be patient.

"I want to know what's going on. Why are all those needles by my grandmother's bed?"

"I was going to check her coags after dinner."

"You have *two* tubes."

"Well, sometimes the vacuum doesn't work on one."

"And number nineteen butterflies. What do you think you're doing?"

"Drawing blood." I was in no mood to argue about the size needles one should use to draw blood. "The floor's out of twenty-ones."

"I don't want you sticking my grandmother with a god-damn number nineteen, understand?"

"I understand, but —"

"I'll draw it," he said. "Just do me a favor, don't ever stick her with nineteens."

"Be my guest." I set the receiver down. Exhaustion had settled permanently in my psyche, as much a part of my equipment as the stethoscope draped around the back of my neck, the rubber tourniquet tied to my clipboard, or the beeper clipped to my belt like a pistol. The elevators were always on the blink, my feet hurt, I was aching for sleep: these were givens. But few nights on call went by without a page from Ernie. He generally managed to interrupt dinner. Not that it was much to interrupt. I looked around at the vending machines. The cafeteria was closed for the summer — an economy move — and no one seemed to care that the interns lived on stale sandwiches. I finished mine as slowly as possible, praying that Ernie, with his worn-down shoe soles and graying hair, would be off my floor by the time I got back.

My grandmother needs suctioning. Tell the nurse to get in here and change the sheets. Why isn't the head of the bed up? Didn't you stop the gent and carb yet? Christ, her BUN's been rising for a week. Where are the calorie counts recorded? How come *you* never know what's going on here?

Mrs. Jonas wasn't even my patient. She belonged to Rick, the other intern on my floor. Rick wrote the orders every morning, Rick made decisions with our junior resident and our attending. My job was just to keep the old lady breathing until morning rounds. Don't let her bleed out, culture her for fevers, bang her chest if she arrests. Simple.

When I got upstairs Ernie was gone. So were the syringes, the butterfly needles, the two blue-topped test tubes I had placed by the old lady's bed half an hour before. I assumed that meant Ernie had drawn her blood. Which was fine with me.

I looked at the old lady lying there in bed, scarcely rattling the phlegm in her throat. It was amazing to me that she breathed. She looked — and this is no exaggeration — like one of the mummies in the British Museum, unwrapped. Toothless, her face was ravaged and desiccated, its skin tough as papyrus. Her limbs were leather-wrapped sticks, except for the artificial prosthesis that bulged from one hip. Infection kept the wound from closing. When she spoke, which was rarely, it was in German. Ernie understood; I didn't want to. I knew enough. The broken hip had only started it all. It was set properly, scientifically. Then came complications. A wound infection. Pulmonary embolus. Pneumonia. This week we wondered if she had had a myocardial infarction — a heart attack. She was the disaster case every intern dreads, a guarantee of three hours' work a night. And Ernie took an hour more.

Ernie came back later that night. I had worked up three new admissions and was exhausted.

"I want you to listen to her breathe," he said. I followed him into her room. The old lady was sleeping peacefully, a bit of rattling in her throat, nothing more. "Listen! That's a disgrace! Why isn't she getting suctioned?"

"Ask the nurse."

"I did. She says she's the only nurse on the floor and I should talk to you."

"Well, your grandmother's not in respiratory distress." My anger flared, then burst. I just wanted sleep, never mind a little phlegm in an old lady's throat. It was two A.M. I looked at Ernie; he was exhausted. He had his own service downstairs, and wasn't even on tonight. He was a jerk for staying here, no question about it. But in a way I admired him. He had courage. He was not afraid to touch her or examine her or draw her blood, and he nursed her as closely as I imagine John Keats, doctor as well as poet, nursed his brother Tom when Tom was dying of tuberculosis. I said, "Maybe she needs a private nurse."

"Maybe you should do your job," he replied.

I walked away.

The next morning after rounds I spoke to my resident.

"Can't you get Ernie off my back? It's getting ridiculous. Who cares if I draw blood with a nineteen needle? He has no *sense!*"

"Oh, it's his grandmother," said my resident. "You'd probably do the same thing. I know I would."

"Some grandmother," I said. "I go to draw her blood and she lies there and spits at me. That's the only way I know she's alive."

He shrugged. "Maybe I'll talk to him."

"Do."

He did. Three nights later I was on call, and Ernie paged me again, this time *stat,* to the nursing station. I ran down the hall, and stopped when I saw him.

"What is it, Ernie?"

"I want you to look at her hand."

I went and looked at her hand. Its birdbones were almost lost in a soft purple bag of blood, as they had been since that morning. The technician had not applied pressure long enough after drawing a blood sample. Anyway, it wasn't my fault. It was just one of those things that happen in a hospital and usually don't make any difference. It did seem, though, that more than the usual number of these things were happening to Ernie's grandmother. Rick had calculated the wrong dose of tobramycin. The oxygen had been turned too low when we came by on rounds that morning, the heparin too high. Somehow she had gotten an extra liter of fluid during the day, and now had rales halfway up her back. My resident said doctors and doctors' relatives get worse care than any other patients admitted to a hospital, and I was beginning to see why. I felt kind of sorry for Ernie.

"Is there anything I can do about it?" I said. I held her hand in mine, feeling the soft purplish bag. A grandmother's hand. My grandmother had died only a year before.

"No, nothing," he said. "Just check her later, would you, and make sure she has the mask on?"

"All right," I said.

He went off. I stayed in there, looking at her. Tonight she looked more shriveled than ever, further from the realms of existence that the rest of us inhabit. It is no joke to say that most cadavers in anatomy lab are more promising material. I know. I've seen them. On the other hand, it was a kind of miracle that this wizened infant of a nonagenarian was refusing to die but lay there day after day, breathing. She had all the regalia of hopeless extremism — three IVs, a catheter in her bladder, electrodes on her chest attached to a bedside cardiac monitor, a rubber drain in her hip wound. Her hand, which I still held, squeezed mine. Just a grasp reflex, I knew. A release sign, it is called. Release from what? I looked at her shrunken face, almost lost behind an oxygen mask. She was looking at me. Big popping eyes followed me as I moved. I tried to imagine her young but failed. Behind the oxygen mask she was mumbling in German. That was fine. I preferred not

to understand what she was saying. It was easier to give up
that way. But why couldn't Ernie be reasonable?

My own grandmother had been different. With her it was not
a question of doing too much, but of total incapacity to forestall
the arrival of death. I was a medical student at the time. All
the doctors in my family, trained to diagnose and cure, above
all to act, could do nothing. When my grandmother made up
her mind to die, none of us could oppose her. It took little
more than a year for her to win.

She was a child of the West, born in Nebraska in the nine-
ties, when the main streets of Omaha were ruts of dirt, plowed
every day by hooves and iron-hooped wheels, and lined with
high, gloomy wooden houses on either side, shutting out the
prairie. Her mother died soon after childbirth from a birth-
related infection. Her father was a lawyer who didn't give
much thought to his baby girl but wanted to be a man about
town, so far as one could be in Omaha at the turn of the
century. So my grandmother was raised by her grandfather,
an immigrant, a politician, once telegrapher to Abraham Lin-
coln and founder of a newspaper, the *Omaha Bee*.

What always struck me most was not that he had always
been on the wrong side in politics, in favor of the banks and
railroads and against the Populists, but that he had done business with Buffalo Bill. As an entrepreneur, he was smart enough
to get a cut in the production of the *Wild West Show* when it
came to Omaha, and the young girl he cared for, his grand-
daughter, had her photograph taken sitting on Buffalo Bill's
knee. Nothing in the rest of her life would match this event.
Buffalo Bill gave her a tobacco pouch, a piece of Indian bead
and leatherwork that is still among the family's possessions.
We grandchildren used to take the stiff and dry relic for show-
and-tell, knowing we were made a part of history by touching

it, and that our wrinkled, pleasant grandmother who invited
us over to watch TV after school and made Boston coolers,
floats of root beer and vanilla ice cream, and read mystery
novels and Shakespeare, was no ordinary woman: she was
history.

She was a cranky, mean, depressed, incontinent, impatient,
forgetful woman before she died. For two years her life was a
constant misery. In William Carlos Williams's poem "The Last
Words of My English Grandmother," I see the woman my
grandmother became.

> There were some dirty plates
> and a glass of milk
> beside her on a small table
> near the rank disheveled bed
>
> Wrinkled and nearly blind
> she lay and snored
> rousing with anger in her tones
> to cry for food
>
> Gimme something to eat —
> They're starving me —

Here are the traces of long misery; the observer is familiar
with this scene, which as a doctor he has often seen before,
and he can enumerate the elements of decay. But he pulls away.
Though he is a grandson, her illness makes them unrelated,
and though he is a doctor he cannot cure. She dies on the way
to the hospital.

> What are all those
> fuzzy-looking things out there?
> Trees? Well, I'm tired
> of them and rolled her head away.

And that is the end of the poem. Fortunately for Williams, poet and doctor, the death came quickly, mercifully, leaving him, the survivor, free to mourn.

My grandmother died slowly. She starved herself. It was a nonviolent, gentlewoman's choice. But it was mercilessly slow. The stroke came first. Thirty years before, she had lost her breasts to cancer, a catastrophe that first threatened, then was forgotten. It never recurred. At sixty-five she went around the world, at seventy she revised her cookbook of diets for patients with heart disease for a second edition, and for another decade she baked innumerable birthday cakes for sixteen grandchildren and played bridge twice a week.

The stroke, which was mild, left her with a droop on one side of her face, a tremor in one arm. But it ruined shopping for her, because people stared. And it ruined reading, or what was left of it. Cataracts had already forced her to large-print books, driving her away from Shakespeare and to thick mysteries, with only a paragraph of intrigue per page. The stroke ruined book-holding and page-turning and snacks of cookies and sweet tea between chapters.

Slowly, she stopped everything. The books my mother brought from the library sat in thick, plastic dust-jacketed piles on the dining room table. She ate less and less. She wanted to die.

The family conferred, consultations of one doctor with another. Why would such a small event as a mild stroke affect her so profoundly? It did not take long to find a medically sound answer: depression. And informally, her treatment was planned. Physical therapy was indicated for her stroke-weakened limbs; she needed better medication for her heart condition; activities with other elderly Jewish ladies at Menorah Park; and to help with feedings, a live-in nurse.

How much better off we were, modern and scientific, coping with our problem than John Keats, poorly and reluctantly trained as a surgeon and apothecary, who tried to nurse his brother Tom back to health. All Keats could do was observe.

"Tom is not up yet — I cannot say he is better."

"Poor Tom is no better tonight — I am affraid [sic] to ask him what message I shall send from him —"

"Tom has spat a leetle blood this afternoon, and that is rather a damper — but I know — the truth is there is something real in the World."

At times he hopes. "I think Tom has been rather better these few last days — he has been less nervous."

And finally, the day of Tom's death, in a letter to his sister Fanny, Keats writes, "He is in a very dangerous state — I have scar[c]e any hopes of him."

To save Tom, Keats needed INH and rifampin, antituberculous drugs. One might speculate that these drugs could have saved John Keats, too, from a miserable, premature death in Italy, where Joseph Severn nursed him, as Keats had nursed Tom. But why waste time on the past, when the best treatment was inadequate? We had the advantages of scientific medicine, and we were all doctors — surely we could solve this problem.

Rehabilitation was the key, said my father, the cardiologist. She was lonely, my mother, the pediatrician, believed. She needed to get out of the house, to get more stimulation, thought my uncle, the internist. I wondered whether her doctor was on top of the medical problems.

A round-the-clock nurse was engaged at considerable expense. My mother got Talking Books. My father spoke with her doctor. Everyone thought there must be some sort of geriatric program in which she could get involved.

But nothing came of it.

"I don't like that *girl*," said my grandmother. The "girl" was a sixty-year-old practical nurse with grandchildren of her own. "I can't eat what she cooks. She drinks, I can smell it on her breath. She doesn't come when I ring for her. Slow as molasses. Honestly," she said to my mother, "can't you find somebody else?"

Another nurse was hired. She quickly became sullen and slow, sitting for hours on a stool in the kitchen, looking out at the back garden, and quit after a month. Still another arrived, then a series of calm, dignified, middle-aged nurses appeared, only to grow angry and quit or be fired. None would do. One cheated on her taxes, another was caught going through the silver, and none of them could make my grandmother comfortable, or get to her before whatever bodily urge she felt became unbearable.

She didn't want any part of Menorah Park.

"I don't know those old people. What do I have to say to them?"

"Nellie shouldn't have to go out," said my grandfather. "It's too hard on her." As for physical therapy, that was too hard on her as well. And the medications — well, she had been going to the same doctor for years, and he thought everything was all right. He didn't see the need to change anything.

The Talking Books, the food, the nurses, even the color television her three children had bought, were too much. "Oh, *heavens,* leave me alone!" She sat in the soft leather armchair in the dining room, by the swinging door that led to the pantry, with an aluminum walker before the chair, pads underneath her to keep things dry, untouched food on the tray by her side, along with letters, postcards, magazines, books my mother continued to check out of the library for her, all untouched. What she did touch was a little silver bell she used to call the nurse, and this she would reach for again and again, often barely letting the nurse leave the room before ringing again.

Only one of her three children did not become a doctor.

When he was fifteen my uncle Ed was given a motion picture camera and, from his first shaky footage of the 1939 World's Fair, has done little but make movies. He never left Ohio, though, or medicine either, really, for his films are about aphasia and heart disease and health programs in industry. He took movies of birthdays, holidays, anniversaries. One June, Ed shot footage of his parents, my grandparents, at their fiftieth anniversary. It shows my grandmother, a few months before her death, thin and irritable, pushed from anniversary cake in the dining room to a reception in the living room, to group pictures in the back yard, by the full-blooming foxglove and the thick foliage of pear and apple trees. It is a bright, muggy Ohio summer day. Every so often she attempts a smile, but mostly it is the irritability that one sees, or an unpleasant expression, as if she had just drunk something very bitter.

She died that fall.

I was in California then, working in the county hospital in the smog-bound valley, doing surgery. My resident was a greyhound-thin, young, balding man with a haggard face and cancer of the stomach. His unfair disease had curdled him and made him mean. I think the only things he loved were his hunting dogs, Blue and Brandy, and he spent whatever time he could lying in his duck blind on the bay with a shotgun in his hands, waiting for birds.

I told him there had been a death in my family and I had to go back to Ohio for the funeral.

"Who died?" he said.

"My grandmother."

"Your *grand*mother? You have to leave for that?"

"Well, my family . . ."

He shrugged. "Just let somebody know if you come back before the end of the month."

On the plane back East, I practiced surgical knots, looping

strands of triple-O black nylon to the back of the seat ahead of me, whipping the threads around with one- and two-handed knots, until the suture ends were too short to tie. I scarcely looked out at the country over which we were flying; instead I thought of layers of skin, fat, fascia, a succession of muscle fibers set at a bias to one another, leading down into a red narrow opening of belly, which soon after opening began filling up with blood. I stood to one side, holding the liver back with a flat metal retractor. My resident had been in a sarcastic mood. "God damn it," he said, "I can't see a damn thing. Come on, pull! Pull on that retractor. You want to go to your grandmother's funeral? Then you better pull until you fasciculate!"

Throughout the service I kept thinking of the operation and trying to figure out why my fingers were still so slow tying knots. Only later would I discover that my technique, furious as it might be, was entirely wrong. I wore the blue suit from my high school graduation and stood in front of the chapel, greeting my grandparents' friends and collecting signatures in a condolence book. I was dazed, exhausted, no more in Ohio than my grandmother herself.

The eulogy was given by our rabbi, a large man who did not know my grandmother. She was not a religious woman, but had been known to the previous rabbi, a famous Zionist and orator, father of the one who stood before us now, searching for words. She had outlived the Zionist, though.

After the service, everyone drove over to my grandfather's house for a reception. The place had been straightened up and the dining room table pushed up to the front window and covered with a tablecloth and food. Two black women in white uniforms, like nurses', were serving punch. People grouped around my grandfather, who looked frail and stunned, small in his baggy suit. There were doctors all over. My family, his old colleagues and friends. My grandmother's leather chair had been stripped of its waterproof cover, and the tray by its side had been removed. But the silver bell and a stack of tapes, not yet returned to the company that rented Talking Books, had been moved to the buffet and apparently forgotten there. The leather pillows of the chair were still indented by my grandmother's shape, as if her weight, invisibly, remained there.

Then I felt like crying. Until that time it had been as if there were no death. What had occurred at the synagogue was not a funeral but a memorial service, and there had been no casket, no mention of a cemetery or headstone, no evidence that the woman who was being remembered had been alive only two days before. The presence of death was an accident, embarrassing as a drunken guest or a family quarrel, something to turn away from in silence, to attempt to ignore. So many doctors and no cure.

The Anatomy Lab was fresh in my mind. The smell of formalin, the big plastic zippered bags like the ones we used to see on the news from the Vietnam front. A dozen cadavers lay in that room; two dozen students worked on them, in a year making lifelike shapes into horrors of nerves, vessels and bones. No wonder, as my grandmother failed, I did not want to know the details — no wonder I did not care to hear that she was in the hospital again, or want to visit her there. The smell of formalin from Anatomy Lab penetrated our rubber gloves and permeated our hair; we frequently joked about why we were standing with scalpels and forceps while these others lay in their bags. Why them, not us? Later we became comfortable to the point of sacrilege, drinking Cokes and eating birthday cake before opening our dissecting manuals and the zippered bags. But that was no more rational than the fear of touching we'd had at first. What remained, I suppose, was panic, a fear of getting too near to the otherness of death, which the doctor feels almost as strongly as he feels an attraction toward, a fascination with, disease. On Tuesday, August 18, 1818, John Keats wrote to his sister Fanny:

> I did not intend to have returned to London so soon but have a bad sore throat from a cold I caught in the island of Mull: therefore I thought it best to get home as soon as possible and went on board the Smack from Cromarty . . .
>
> Tom has not been getting better since I left London and for the past fortnight has been worse than ever — he has been getting a little better for these two or three days . . .
>
> — all I can say now is that your Letter is a very nice one without fault and that you will hear from or see in a few days if ~~my~~ his throat will let him,
>
> Your affectionate Brother
JOHN.

The last sentence is ungrammatical — there is no object for the verbs. From whom will Fanny hear? More revealingly, Keats crosses out "my" and writes "his." Whose throat is it? Who is the patient? It is likely that this sore throat is the beginning of tuberculosis for John Keats, who soon after will himself cough drops of bright red arterial blood. "I cannot be deceived in that colour; that drop is my death warrant. I must die." This is Lord Houghton's report of Keats's reaction. But Keats, in a letter to his sister, admits to saying only "This is unfortunate." Is this the essence of the doctor's fear? Does a related illness, the illness of a relative, presage the doctor's own death? Behind his starched white coat the doctor is terrified that instead of the student of disease he will become the disease itself. No wonder doctors are not permitted to treat their own families or themselves.

I do not remember much more about the day of my grandmother's memorial service, except that my grandfather looked every one of his eighty-nine years, and that after a while everyone went out back to the garden, and stood on wet grass before a pear tree loaded with hard, small fruit, and posed for family snapshots.

The next day I went back to California and to surgery. It was a wonderful month, and for a while I was sure I would become a surgeon. Every day I awoke at five A.M. and hurried to the hospital, where I could hardly wait to put on my greens and scrub up to my elbows with yellow-soaped sponges, then rush into cool, tiled rooms where a gown would be pulled on me and tied and tight gloves snapped onto my hands, and then lean up against the operating table, holding retractors and peering into body cavities, just waiting for my chance to get hold of forceps and needle-holder and bring skin back together. My knots came fast and tight. The skin I sewed met in smooth lines. Even my cancerous resident stopped saying his dogs were smarter than I and asked if I was interested in doing more months of surgery. I did do more surgery after that, cardiac surgery, and loved it. But by June, and the end of the rotation, I was sick — a variety of minor complaints, nothing that sleep and regular meals would not alleviate. When I got better I realized that I had cracked more chests, peered at more diseased hearts and sewed more skin than I would ever care to remember. Only a long time later did I realize that I had despised the whole experience, and that it had all been a kind of mourning. I wanted to make up for all that was lost.

The night before she died, Mrs. Jonas, as always, spat at me as I drew her blood. I crouched at her side, careful to advance the needle so it punctured only one side of the slippery vein, then coursed along inside. No spittle hit me — she could only purse her lips and blow air through them. But the intent was clear.

"Okay, Mrs. Jonas, take it easy," I said, holding her hand.

I did feel relieved. She had been declared NTBR — not to be resuscitated if her heart stopped. I did not know all the details, whether the chief resident had talked to Ernie, or whether Ernie and his family had just gotten tired of it all. But I did know there were no more emergencies.

I finished drawing her blood and put pressure on the puncture site for five minutes. I didn't want it to bleed, not with Ernie around. The old lady stared at me as if I had just shot her in the heart. I went off to do my fever rounds before going to sleep in one of the empty patient rooms.

When I woke up it was already light out, and a nurse was shaking me.

"Mrs. Jonas's pressure is still down."

"What?"

"I told you before it had dropped. Remember?"

Did I remember?

"What is it now?"

"It was sixty over forty. Now it's fifty over zero."

"Oh, Jesus."

I got up. It was 6:30 A.M., almost time for rounds, the hour that old ladies die. Mrs. Jonas was flat on her back in bed, motionless as Nefertiti. Her skin was gray. I felt her wrist, just above the purple bag of blood, but there was no pulse. I felt her neck. A beat, then another, then nothing. So life fades. I looked at her for a long time. I pounded her chest once, then again. Nothing. I put down the head of the bed, turned up the IV all the way, then realized, almost as an afterthought, that she was not breathing. Should I breathe her? I looked out the window at the river below, at rush-hour traffic crossing the bridge and at three tugboats pushing a barge upstream. NTBR meant don't breathe her. But still . . . My own grandmother had faded off, too; she had awakened only at the last moment to call her husband, my grandfather. "Harold! Harold, please, I need you!" When he and my mother came back into the room — they had been on their way to the elevator — she was dead.

Eventually I turned off the IV. She was, after all, NTBR. Enough was enough.

I caught Ernie in the hall, just a few minutes before morning rounds, and when I stopped him I thought he was going to punch me in the face. But instead he looked almost apologetic.

"How did it happen?" he asked.

I told him, more or less.

He said something I could not make out.

"What?"

"Thank you," he said. I looked at him. "I . . . look, I'm going to go in and see her. And then call my family. Look, could you just make sure the papers are filled out early, so we can get her to the funeral home?"

"Sure," I said. Then I went off to rounds. It was not until 6:00 P.M., after I had written all my notes and was ready to leave the hospital, that Ernie paged me.

"You the intern?"

"Yeah, what?" Then I remembered. "Oh, damn it, I forgot! I'm sorry, Ernie."

"That's all right. I know how it gets," he said.

When I came downstairs to the front desk, to fill out the death papers, he was not there. I leaned up against a counter and began to sign my name to the forms for the city of New York, on which were typed the name and address of Gretchen Jonas and the causes of death.

> *Respiratory Arrest* occurring as a complication of
> *Myocardial Infarction* occurring as a complication of
> *Pulmonary Embolus* occurring as a complication of
> *Hip Fracture.*

"That's no good," said the woman at the desk when I handed it to her.

"What do you mean?"

"You have to use a black pen."

I looked at my name, written in blue ink.

"Do you have a black pen? I'll trace over it."

"I can't do that. The city won't accept it."

"I'll take the responsibility."

"You can't. No way. You have to write the whole thing over."

"Oh, for Christ's sake."

"Or you can wait for the forms to be typed again. That'll take until tomorrow."

"I swear, we spend more time here with the dead patients than the live ones," I said.

She gave me the forms. I remembered what Keats wrote after Tom died, in a letter to his other brother, George. "During poor Tom's illness I was not able to write and since his death the task of beginning has been a hindrance to me."

"Do you have a black pen?" I said.

She slapped it down on the counter, with that peculiar fury New Yorkers have when they consider themselves imposed on.

"Thanks a lot," I said. I began to write.

The Gray Ones

SHE WAS FOURTEEN, just a kid, and it was already in her by the time I inherited her from the intern going off service. He had not left an off-service note in the chart, however, and even the admission note was incomplete, because after coming in at 2:00 A.M. she'd gone directly to the operating room. She'd come from Georgia in a private Lear Jet chartered by her father, and brought the kidney, floating in an electrolyte solution inside an ice chest, with her. Later she'd show pictures of herself in the airport in Atlanta, a cheerful round-faced girl in designer jeans and a fringed shirt, her pupils blazing red from the flashbulb. On the floor between her cowboy boots sat the red and white ice chest, the kind you usually see full of beer at a football game. But on rounds the first morning all I saw was a beautiful, pallid young girl, asleep. She looked like someone I knew.

She moaned with pain when we pulled off the dressing. There it was, on the left side, between navel and the ridge of hipbone, beneath an incision angled like an appendectomy scar. The cut was like a mouth sewn shut; skin bulged up around it, as though there was a fist inside, pushing out.

"How's her output?" asked the Renal fellow, Raphael. Raphael, a gawky ex-hippie from Bronxville, was wearing a flannel shirt that was half untucked and muddy lumberjack boots. He had scraggly long black hair in a ponytail and tobacco-stained fingers and seemed unaware of how wild he looked — or totally indifferent to it. He pulled the chart from my hands. "Incredible! Four hours post-op and she's already put out a liter."

"Is that a good sign?" I asked.

"Does it mean she won't reject? I don't know. But I've never seen one open up so fast. It's amazing." He hefted the collecting bag before us; it was connected to a plastic tube that went to the Foley catheter in her bladder. Urine tinged with blood poured through the tubing as we watched.

"I tell you, if anyone deserves to have their transplant work it's this kid," Raphael said. She'd been on dialysis two years, he explained, and had already had pericarditis twice and high blood pressure and severe bone disease, not to mention the anemia and slowed growth that all kids on dialysis had. She had a rare tissue type, and so many antibodies to foreign tissue, too, that it had been nearly impossible to cross match her with the kidneys of potential donors. But finally a kidney had come, from a young man whose skull had been crushed in a motorcycle accident in the Florida panhandle.

"How are you at starting lines?" Raphael inquired.

"Pretty good. Why?"

"Well, you're going to have to get daily lytes and creatinines for quite a while. She gave the other intern a hard time. Wouldn't even let him draw blood."

"Great. That's what I love about kids."

"Hey, Robin!" He shook the girl until her eyes opened. Her first half-yawn was stopped abruptly by the pain in her belly, and then she was awake. "Meet your new doctor."

Drowsily, she looked me over in such a way that I could tell she had had a lot to do with doctors and didn't like them much. I could see the battles ahead.

"Hello," she said. "How's my kidney?"

"Fine," I told her. Now, too, I saw why she looked familiar; it was her coloring — the fairness of her skin, scattered with freckles, and her hair, which was curly, short, so blond it was almost white, and the even pallor of her eyelashes and lips. She was the kind who must rely on blood for coloring, who chaps and burns on an overcast day at the beach. Before medical school, when I was living in San Francisco and trying to be Frank O'Connor, I knew someone with that coloring — a woman who would drive me up in the Berkeley hills in her boyfriend's Triumph — who used to say that when she closed her eyes her face disappeared. And when her green eyes closed, it did.

"What you do today," said Raphael, "is draw her bloods — send them *stat* — make sure she's on the list for a renal scan, and follow her I's and O's real close. And write for her steroid taper. Got it?"

"Yeah, sure. What's her name again?"

"Robin. And one more thing. Don't stick yourself when you're getting her bloods. She's got hepatitis."

I have to admit that I never much liked taking care of kids. When I was a medical student, working on that Pediatrics ward in the county hospital with infants with irreparable defects in their hearts, and kids whose skulls were fractured in car accidents and who would never wake up, and freaky inhuman creatures with wide-set eyes and low ears and dull, reptilian expressions, babies who would never assemble a thought, it became too much for me. It got me in a way that an old man dying of congestive heart failure or lung cancer didn't get me. I could handle the old guys; a good number of them had ruined themselves, and anyway, they'd lived. But not the kids. Try sticking a skinny little butterfly needle into the chubby wrist of a three-year-old and you'll see what I mean. You hurt them; they hate you. It's not just babies, either, it's kids, ten and twelve and fourteen. You're still part of the disease, the torture. You want to give up and cry with them, and if you feel that way you could never be much of a pediatrician. The only part I liked was talking to the mothers.

So I avoided children. It wasn't difficult; there were more than enough other things to learn in medical school, and it was not anything that would be noticed, much less commented on, by anyone. As an intern in New York City, I made the same choice. It was either two months of Pediatrics, or I could risk hepatitis and spend the time on the dialysis and transplantation unit, the Renal Service. I chose Renal.

And here, the first morning on rounds, I made an ironic discovery: of my half dozen or so patients, three were kids. Next to Robin, whose kidney failure had come from a congenital malformation and repeated infections, there was Tommy Kramer, a twelve-year-old boy with Henoch-Schönlein purpura, a rare disease. In the bed across from Robin was Don Green, a fourteen-year-old who looked six. As a baby he'd had radiation therapy for a tumor in his belly; the tumor disappeared, but his kidneys gradually shrank and failed. The fourth kid in the room, not my patient, was Karen O'Connell, with lupus erythematosus. The four of them were in a room together, separated from other patients, not because of their age but because they'd had transplants and were subject to their own sorts of complications and diseases.

We circled the room, feeling the fist-sized lumps of foreign tissue in their bellies to make sure they were not tender or enlarged, which could signify rejection; we picked up collecting bags full of urine; we put stethoscopes to rib cages to listen for the crackling of pneumonia; we searched inside mouths for yeast infections; we palpated the snakelike fistulas in their arms for the whirring that meant blood still flowed. If the transplants failed, they'd be used again.

They were strange kids. Disease had joined them into a family, made them all of a kind. Not only were they all small and baby-faced and fat in the middle and thin in the arms and legs, not only did they all have fistulas snaking up their arms, but they shared a certain tinge of skin. Clay dust might have been rubbed into them, or lead-colored blood might run in their veins. Robin was less dull than the others, but I don't know why — maybe an accident of chemistry, maybe she hadn't been on dialysis as long. In her fresh complexion the gray of uremia and the yellow of hepatitis were scarcely visible.

But the kids shared more than coloration. There was something odd in the way they watched us, the way they lay in bed, as if so accustomed to spending their days there and feeling sick and seeing doctors come by that they could not imagine life any other way. And they talked like doctors.

"What's my creatinine today?"

"My output's two thousand three hundred cc's and yesterday it was three thousand. Does that mean I'm rejecting?"

"How much longer am I getting Imuran?"

"My blood pressure's high. Do you think we should go up on my hydralazine?"

"Is my foot-drop going to get better now I'm off dialysis?"

Raphael waved their questions aside. "Give him a break. He hasn't had a chance to read your charts yet."

And we went to finish rounds. There were twenty other patients to see. I had an old poet with diabetes and kidney failure, a businessman with uncontrollably high blood pressure and kidney failure, an African diplomat's wife with a mysterious rash and kidney failure (both probably caused by African doctors), and a lady in her fifties who had been on dialysis a long time and was now so demented we were going to let her die.

At the end we came to the Dialysis Center, a long room with a dozen beds, each occupied by a man or woman in street clothes, and a dozen machines. Out of ashen arms came plastic tubes, surprisingly bright with blood, which curled toward the coils and tanks of the dialysis machines. Some patients were watching the televisions suspended overhead, others read the *Times* or *The New Yorker* or were spared from the general din by the foam earphones of their Walkman tape players. And still others scratched themselves, rhythmically and slowly, as if they did it by the hour. They were mostly outpatients, Raphael said, and they came in shifts, day and night. The room had the air of a bus terminal or a twenty-four-hour variety store, a place constantly occupied, year after year, whose floor can be scrubbed continually but never cleaned, and where the air itself gets exhausted from uninterrupted breathing. We had only two patients here: a drug addict from Jersey and an ancient, comatose man shipped in from a nursing home to keep his daughters happy. We examined them hurriedly — it was no place to linger.

On our way out, we passed a little boy, three or four at most and already gray as an old nickel, being led in by his mother. When he saw us, massed in white pants and coats like one many-headed ghost, he screamed with terror and broke from his mother. He ran down the corridor, chased by two wide-hipped nurses, and was almost off the ward before they caught him. We could still hear his screaming after they carried him back in.

"Don't stick me there. They did that yesterday. It still hurts. No, not there, either. I don't want to get a scar. If you do it on my hand it hurts too much. And there, if you do it there, I'll get a bruise . . ."

Unfortunately, Robin had awakened when I came to push medications and draw blood.

"What about the other arm?"

She eyed me with disdain.

"You can't go on that side, that's my *fistula* arm. There's too much risk of infection. Don't you know that?"

"Of course. Well, I *do* have to get your blood. Do you have any suggestions?"

She gazed down at her arm. It was soft, scattered with blond hairs so fine they were almost invisible, and its perfection was marred only by the tape of the intravenous line and a small bruise in the crook of the elbow where blood had been taken last night. If not for the failure of her kidneys, the perfect limb of a pubescent Daisy Buchanan. A Sunbelt version of Daisy Buchanan, but nonetheless American, one sent to Aspen to ski, to Cancún for sun, destined for a small college in a Confederate state, for sufficient but not dangerous learning, and for marriage to a man who could guarantee more of the same. You could see how dialysis botched the whole plan.

"How about there?" she suggested.

I put my tourniquet around her arm, and a vein popped up right below her finger.

"Okay."

"Are you using a number twenty-three butterfly?" she said. "Otherwise it hurts too much."

"Yes, I'm using a number twenty-three."

I pulled back slowly on the syringe.

"Is my kidney really working okay?"

"It's fine. You've put out two or three liters already."

"It is? You know, I carried it myself, all the way from Georgia. I could have had the transplant in Miami, but we came here especially because of the RPGG. I'm going to get that, aren't I?"

I had never heard of it.

"It's experimental. My dad thinks it's the best stuff. He talked with the doctors at every transplant program in the country before I came here. And he read all the studies."

"He's a doctor?"

"No, he's a businessman. Aren't you done yet?"

"Yeah. Hold on here, okay? Just put some pressure with your thumb."

There's no question but that hemodialysis prolongs life. Without it, a person with kidney failure would die in a few days. Yet it is expensive and painful and disabling. Surprisingly few people on dialysis are able to work; surprisingly many are abandoned by their husbands or wives; surprisingly many become apathetic and listless.

Like many other technologies in medicine, dialysis is at once sophisticated and crude. It goes only halfway. It is applied imperfectly to diseases that are only partially understood, treating the effects of disease but not the cause. It palliates but does not cure. Similarly, the treatment of cancer patients with chemotherapy and radiation shrinks the tumor but poisons the body; and the coronary artery bypass detours the obstruction but does not slow the clogging of vessels. Even insulin, which saves diabetics, does not prevent some of them from going blind or losing limbs to poor circulation.

With dialysis, the problem is the imperfect way in which it substitutes for the kidneys. With current technology, the waste product urea cannot be removed from the blood. From excess urea, or uremia, comes a host of complications — anemia, infections, pericarditis, atherosclerosis, metabolic bone disease, chemical abnormalities, encephalopathies (disturbances of consciousness, including irreversible dementia) and peripheral neuropathies. These alone can make life miserable. And every time dialysis is done, needles must be stuck in the shunt or fistula for access to the circulation, with a risk of clotting, infection and bleeding that is small each time but significant over a lifetime. A review in *Kidney International* concluded that the incidence of complications in hemodialysis is "difficult to answer with an exact percentage," but

> the complication rate in the young patient is sufficiently high, however, that transplantation should be seriously considered as a means of restoring normal renal function. Of course, one must consider complications from that therapy as well.

That afternoon we went to Radiology and looked at Robin's first renal scan. Raphael should have known better, I guess, from having seen other transplant patients, but still he got all enthusiastic. It was something in Robin, I think, because I felt it, too.

"Look at that; look at that flow." He jabbed his bony right forefinger, with a jagged yellowed nail, toward the fluorescent panel on which hung two pieces of film. The one on the left side showed four separate frames scattered with black dots. "See, there's the dye going in, there's the descending aorta, and there in the left inguinal region, there's the kidney. Look at the way that sucker lights up."

We all looked — the other residents and the radiologist and I.

"And look over here." He rubbed his finger against the film on the right. "Excretion's just as good. I'm telling you, I've never seen it that good before."

"I have," said the radiologist. "And sometimes those are the ones that reject the worst."

"She won't," said Raphael.

For three days Robin's kidney poured out urine, filling the bag so that the nurse would have to come in and empty it every few hours. Robin would lie in bed, surrounded by her

stuffed animals and dozens of get-well cards from her classmates in Atlanta and her aunt and uncle in San Clemente and
her camp in Wyoming and the kids with whom she went to
Mexico in sixth grade, and new deliveries of flowers would
come to the nurses' station every day, so irises and carnations
and roses in cellophane filled her corner of the room, enough
flowers all told for a Kentucky Derby winner and a mobster's
funeral combined. Her parents, a pleasant, prematurely gray
mother and a tensely jovial dad, were there from eight in the
morning to eleven at night. Her father was a potbellied guy
who favored wide-wale electric green corduroy pants and
sweaters that buttoned down the front. He looked as if he'd
feel much more comfortable on a golf course, but he spent his
days reading through Xeroxed articles from the *New England
Journal of Medicine* and *Kidney International,* so he could
give us advice. Every time I came into the room, Dad would
want to have a conference about the latest developments. He'd
have her urine output totaled to the last cc, and know her last
five blood pressures, and he'd want her creatinine as soon as
it came off the computer from the lab.

"What do you think?" he'd ask. Robin's mother would look
up and smile with her mouth closed.

"Oh, it looks good," I'd say. "Of course, you can never tell
for sure, you can't predict. But for the moment, everything
looks fine."

She was the queen of the room. The other kids struggled to
put out a liter of urine a day, and she did it every other hour.
Tommy Kramer was rejecting his kidney — a gift from his
older sister — and he would get up and walk around the room,
his oversized feet flapping, ungainly as rubber swimming flip-
pers. He'd hoist himself up on the side of his bed and sit mo-
rosely, working a pencil into his drawing of the Empire State
Building as Robin chattered. Then he'd disappear off to dialysis for half a day and come back dull and drawn, and lay

his sketch pad aside. Across from Robin, Don Green hunched into his bed; only one get-well card, from his mother in Yonkers, protected him from the invasion of flowers and cards that marched from Robin's side across the window ledge. And diagonally from Robin, round Karen O'Connell began talking nonsense. At night, after her family left, she wandered down the hall, her Foley bag dragging on the floor behind her, IV bottles crashing. And Robin's creatinine plummeted.

I came in every morning with tubes for blood, butterfly IVs, syringes of medication, and waited, irritated and hurried, while she chose a spot for me to stick. But then I found myself staying there longer than I needed to, talking about her horse out in the country or what she should see in Manhattan before she went back, or whatever.

Then, on the fourth day, the urine stopped as if dammed up inside. Her temperature rose. When I came in with my needles and syringes and the metal boxes that held blood culture bottles, I found her sitting forward in bed, eyes puffy, elbows squeezed into her sides. Her father leaned against the window ledge, poring over his reprints.

"I'm rejecting, aren't I?" she said.

I said that we weren't sure yet; she might just have an infection.

"Why did this have to happen? It was going so well. It was the best you guys ever saw, that's what you said, isn't it?"

"Robin, we just don't know yet."

"I *am* rejecting. I can feel it. Touch my kidney — see how big it is?" She held my hand in her fat little-girl hand with chipped pink nail polish and a clammy palm, and she set my hand on her lower belly, atop the incision, where I could feel the bulge of the graft. It was almost as if I fingered the bruised, swollen thing itself, battered by angry blood that swirled through it, a dangerous, foreign object, under siege.

"What are you going to *do?*" she screamed. Tommy laid

down his sketch pad and looked across at us, with a kind of satisfaction, it seemed. "What if I lose it? I don't want to lose it. Do *something!*"

"Calm down, Robin, it'll be okay," I said.

Her father followed me into the hall.

"You know, in Miami," he said, "the way they treat rejection is —"

"I'll be right back," I said.

I found Raphael in the Conference Room, smoking. There were bits of tobacco in his mustache.

"I really feel sorry for those people."

"What's going on?"

"She's rejecting and they're all frantic."

"Robin?" he asked. He looked startled, as if about to cry. Then he recovered. He dug into his old army knapsack and came up with some grubby sheets of paper, a handout entitled *Immunosuppressive Therapy Following Kidney Transplantation.* "Here we go," he said. " 'Pediatric patient, rejection treatment, first episode.' We can calculate out the doses. How many kilos does she weigh?"

We began the rejection treatment. Nothing grew from the blood cultures. The urine, when it came, was clear, and the X rays were negative; after a few days, her creatinine, which had risen from 0.7 to 3.5, began to fall. Her fevers abated, and her urine output rose from practically nothing to a hundred cc's a day. After two weeks, when her output hit half a liter, her parents, who had been hovering around Robin's bed day and night, hardly going to their hotel room, took a plane back to Atlanta. Robin shone again. She wore a gauzy new nightgown and a bathrobe bright with parrots and jungle foliage. She wrote to her class in Atlanta; she began *Hard Times* for her English class; she interviewed me for her school newspaper — "How did you decide you wanted to be a doctor? Are you especially interested in kidneys?" She would walk down the hall in her bathrobe, the apparatus for her Foley catheter in a shopping bag at her side, her big pale feet in fluffy slippers; she'd come and sit with us in the Intensive Care Unit, or lean over the counter at the nurses' station, until I came by. Then she'd look embarrassed, and after a few minutes she'd say she had something to do in her room and shuffle back down the hall.

Beside her, Tommy Kramer, whose output continued to drop, became accustomed to going to dialysis three times a week; his sister, now out of the hospital, would come and sit silently by his bed. In the other corner, Karen O'Connell became stiff and weird, throwing food off her tray. The other intern did a spinal tap, which grew Listeria meningitides. And Don developed pneumonia.

The room filled with IV bottles, plastic tubing, boxes of gauze pads and plastic syringes, and nurses working extra shifts. We spent half of morning rounds there, passing much of the time around Robin's bed. Raphael would come by every few hours to check her output, I would come into the room to see how she was doing and find the other interns there, holding her blood pressure chart in their hands or sitting in the chair at her bedside. The day she hit eleven hundred cc's, we were all in there, Raphael settling onto the edge of her bed and sighing, as he often did in the mornings before he had his cigarette and coffee.

"I think we've got it licked," he announced.

At midnight that night, when I came by, all the kids were still awake. Tommy and Don were sitting around Karen's bed, sharing a box of chocolate chip cookies brought in by the O'Connells. Robin's curtain was pulled closed.

"You want a cookie?" Karen asked.

"No thanks."

"Your little friend's not feeling so good," she said. The three of them started laughing.

"You'll get fat if you keep eating those," I said.

On the other side of the curtain, Robin lay covered in blankets, so just her face and her knuckles were visible. She was shivering.

"Hi, kid, how're you doing?"

Beneath my hand, her forehead radiated a fury of heat.

"It's happening again," she said. She began crying.

"Damn!" I said, which didn't help much. I sat down on the bed, wondering. How could any surgeon be crazy enough to cut a kidney out of some motorcycle-riding kid who smashed his skull and slice another kid open and sew that kidney inside, and how could anyone be so full of daring and brazen foolishness to think the kidney would work? There was no question about it, the whole idea was insane. And most bizarre and astonishing of all was that often enough the complications passed and the miracle remained. The things *worked.* Anyhow, that was what the textbooks said.

"Look, Robin, don't worry. We'll get it working again. It'll just be a couple of days."

"I don't want to go on dialysis again. I'd rather be dead."

"I said we'll get it working again."

"What are you going to do? Are you going to take more blood? Do you need another X ray? Am I going to get pulsed again?"

"Robin, let me be the doctor, okay?"

"You don't understand. You don't know how horrible it is. I just never know what's going to happen next."

"It's horrible, Robin, I know."

From the nurses' station, I phoned Raphael. His wife answered and said she'd get him. He finally came to the phone and dully said hello, and I told him what was happening. But he seemed drowned in a lubberly morass of sleep, and I had to repeat three times what was going on before he seemed to get it.

"Oh . . . oh, hell," he said. "Look at that . . . that handout again. The second rejection episode in the pediatric patient. It's like last time. Just give twice as much prednisone."

"Isn't that a lot?"

"That's what we give. Got it?"

"Okay."

I could hear his wife in the background, telling him to come back to bed. He sighed.

"Give me a call if you have troubles."

When the medication came up from the pharmacy, in a fifty-cc glass syringe, I brought it into the kids' room and sat beside Robin's bed and pushed it in slowly through a butterfly. She had stopped crying by then, and when I left to work up my new admissions, she was sitting up, staring across the room, where troll-sized Don Green lay tangled in plastic tubing.

At two in the morning, a nurse came into the Conference Room, where I was lying on a cot, trying to sleep.

"What is it?"

"Robin fell out of bed. I think you should see her."

"Fell? How'd that happen?" I reached for my glasses and pulled a white coat over my greens, then stuffed my feet into my shoes and dazedly followed her down the hall.

Robin was already back in bed. Her big pale legs were out of the covers, her nightgown was twisted. She breathed strangely — too loud, forcedly — and there was blood on her arm where the IV had been pulled loose. I shook her and called her name, but she hardly responded. With thumb and forefinger, I opened her eyes, which were unfocused, being-less. A groan, a gutteral animal noise came from her, and suddenly her arms thrashed up at me, driving my glasses against my eyes. I pushed her arms away.

I looked across the bed at the nurse.

"What happened?"

"I don't know. The aide came in to take her temperature and she was on the floor."

Now I saw that her front teeth were slick with blood. And she had a lump at her right temple. For all I knew she could be bleeding into her brain.

Then, unseen strings twitched and jerked her arms, like the limbs of a marionette, and her legs went too. The trembling went through the whole of her, so she arched back into the pillow, gasping, and a horrible, ruddy, inhuman mask replaced her face.

"Oh, Christ!" I said. She was seizing. I stood like a block of wood, as if all the medicine I had ever learned had been shaken loose from my mind, and all I could do was be there forever, watching her choke on her tongue. Finally the nurse pulled a plastic airway from where it was taped to the wall and jammed it into Robin's mouth, twisting it past her teeth.

Then I was able to act.

"She's in status. Get me ten of Valium. Come on, *move*."

I was up with her, worried, all night. Five more times she seized, and I kept pushing medications into her IV lines and sticking needles into veins and arteries for blood and checking the airway and trying to figure out what it was that made her seize. She kept gasping for breath, and the X ray showed a haze of pneumonia rising in her lungs. I pushed antibiotics and anticonvulsants. We transferred her to the Intensive Care Unit, down at the end of the floor. Raphael came in at 3:00 A.M. and stayed two hours, then went back across the street to his wife.

I was in the Conference Room, dazedly staring at her chart, when he arrived for morning rounds.

"There you are," he said. He handed me a paper bag from the deli. "How'd it go after I left?"

Inside the bag was breakfast. I pulled the lid off the cup, tossed it into the bag, and sipped hot, sweet coffee. Then I unwrapped white paper to find a bagel, spread with cream cheese, which was warmed by its nearness to the coffee.

"Poor kid," I said.

"She didn't seize again?"

I shook my head. " 'Course I wouldn't say she's awake yet, either. What do you think did it?"

"Don't know," he said. "Maybe the steroids. Maybe they were just too much for her."

"It doesn't make sense."

"These kids never do," he said. "After they get their transplants, all kinds of strange things happen."

"God, I don't know about this business."

"I tell you," he said, "if I lost my kidneys, I'd stay on dialysis. The transplant's just too much."

"I don't know. I don't know what I'd do." I chewed on the bagel. "Oh! I stuck myself drawing her blood. A goddamn butterfly. I jabbed it right into my thumb."

"Oh boy. You make sure you get your shots. Hyperimmune globulin. One in each cheek. Hurts like hell."

"Shit."

"Let's go in and see her."

I don't remember much of that day, except the drowned look of her face, the slow, confused way she woke, as if the human districts of her brain had been stunned, bombed, blacked out, convulsed into silence, leaving her dazed and crocodilian, aware only of heat and pain and the rush of noises around her. I went down to Employee Health and had my blood drawn and was injected twice, so I went through the rest of the day dizzy and sick from foreign stuff in my veins. I could barely walk back into the unit to check her vacant pupils or push medications. It was evening before she could speak, and nearly a week before she stopped moving like someone whose limbs have fallen asleep. I don't think she ever got it clear in her mind what happened, whether she fell out of bed and then seized, or the other way around. But I do know we did everything possible to save that kidney.

When I say we, I mean not so much the house staff — the residents and interns and fellows — but the faculty members and consultants who generally stay in the background, making brief appearances on the ward two or three times a week and delivering oracular presentations in teaching conferences. Robin's bed was surrounded by them: a few private "slicks" in their five-hundred-dollar suits, a balding marine of a surgeon in his greens and scuffed tennis shoes, a neurologist with a hand-tooled leather case of pins, vials of cinnamon, fancy reflex hammers, tuning forks, pieces of striped cloth. Any hour of day or night I'd come in and see a few of them at the foot of her bed, or examining her belly, or talking transplants and organ banks with her father. Robin was first on the list for renal scans whenever she needed one, and, in desperation, room was found for her on the plasmapheresis machine, which was generally used only for research.

Despite it all, her output slowly dropped. The renal scans showed fewer and fewer dots in the left lower belly, and she began to be sent, twice a week, to the Dialysis Center. She cried every time they wheeled her down the hall, and while she was in there, her mother would be with her, and her father would stand out in the hallway, blankly looking out over the river. And every day I checked the whites of my own eyes, and my own skin, because the shots did not always work.

By the time she was transferred out of Intensive Care, back to her old bed, the room was empty. Don Green's pneumonia had faded and his kidney still worked: he went home to Yonkers. Tommy Kramer's kidney barely kept him off dialysis, yet it did not fail: he went back to Jersey. Even Karen O'Connell's meningitis seemed to resolve: she was sent out to Long Island with her family. For a day or two the other beds were empty, and then because the transplant business was slow, dialysis patients with complications came in. There was one old woman who needed a tuneup of her blood pressure, and two young girls, one with peritonitis and another with a clotted fistula. Robin kept her curtains pulled most of the time.

One afternoon Raphael and I went down to Radiology to check the day's renal scans and found Robin there. The dye had already been injected, and the technician moved the huge sensing apparatus into place over her; on the television monitors by the computer, bursts of dots began to appear.

"It hurts," Robin said. "I can't stand this thing lying on top of me."

I put my hand on her shoulder. The machine was hardly touching her. I said, "Hold still, Robin."

"Come here," said Raphael, and motioned me out of the room. We could still see the monitors, and from a distance you could see where the kidney should be, where on the first days we had seen bright rushes of dots. The radiologist came by.

"You see that — an empty space there?" he said. "Even less absorption than the surrounding area?"

It looked like a hole in the body, like a dark spot in a galaxy, a place too dense for light to escape.

"Yeah, what does that mean?"

"That there's not any blood flow through the kidney. And the kidney's swollen enough that it presses down and there's even less blood flow behind it. It's called a negative image."

"And?"

The technician was guiding the sensing apparatus, a huge metal cylinder, off Robin. She lay there rigidly, as if it hurt just to breathe. The technician wheeled a gurney into the room.

"It's a surgical emergency," the radiologist said. "It's got to come out."

Raphael was already paging the surgeons. In a few minutes they were there.

She was back on the floor by midafternoon, paler than ever, with a white dressing taped over her wound. Her snowy blond hair was spread out on the pillow and her eyes were closed and her cracked lips as pale as her eyelashes, and for a moment it seemed that her face disappeared, and there was only a pink, featureless shell, like the woman I used to know who closed her eyes in a different kind of abandon. But there seemed more gray to Robin now, as if she had been finely coated with dust.

Her father sat in the chair by the side of the bed. He had been crying.

"All I wanted to do was give her a couple of years," he said. "So she wouldn't stop growing yet, so she'd have a chance to be normal for a little while. She's a great kid."

"She is," I said.

"She's a great kid. It's just not fair." And he was crying again.

Within a week she was up again, hobbling back and forth in the hall, playing cards with the nurses — halfheartedly, true, but playing. She had a regular slot at the Dialysis Center by now, and every Monday, Wednesday, and Friday shuffled down the corridor to the room of gray people. One afternoon she even went out with her parents, to Bloomingdale's and to the top of the World Trade Center.

The day she was to leave I went to find her, but her bed was empty and her parents were in her room, throwing flowers into a huge plastic garbage bag. I found her in the Dialysis Center. She was wearing jeans and cowboy boots, and a new shirt from Bloomingdale's, and the needles in her fistula were circulating her bright red blood through the machine. At her side stood Tommy Kramer, looking perhaps a little less gray than he had on the ward. In fact, when I looked from Robin to Tommy, it was disturbing to observe that she was the grayer of the two.

"Hi," said Robin. "You know what, Doctor? Tommy, tell him."

"Karen O'Connell died," Tommy said.

"You're kidding."

"They found her at home and she was dead," said Robin.

"Her mother found her," said Tommy.

"What happened?"

"I don't know. I don't think they know. They found her in the living room and they thought she was asleep but she was dead. Her kidney was still working but she died."

"Tommy's kidney is still working," Robin said.

"No kidding," I said. "That's great."

"And so is Don Green's," Robin said. The dialysis nurse turned some knobs on the machine, and, wearing gloves, pulled the big needles from Robin's arm. Robin put pressure on the wounds with her hand.

"That's two out of four," Robin said.

"That's one way of looking at it," I said.

"What do you mean?" Robin asked. "You know, I'm going to get another one. I'm going to Atlanta until I get back to normal, and then my father's going to put me on the list again. I'm going to come back here, too, next time." She sat up and gingerly swung her legs off the side of the bed. For a moment I was afraid she'd black out. Then the color came back to her face, and she smiled at me, the way I imagine Daisy Buchanan, in her time, must have smiled for Gatsby.

Robin's parents came to the door then, dressed, as always, for the golf course.

"Come on, Robin," said her father.

She eased off the bed, still almost smiling.

"And next time it's going to work," she said.

The Battle
for the Dead

IN THE ROOM with a spectacular view a woman lies open-mouthed, her neck awry. You've come to pronounce her dead. Under your palm her bony chest is warm, but nothing beats under your palm and your fingers feel no movement in the neck, not air or blood. She was old but not that old — just late middle age. Tongue and lips glaze as you watch, and around her eyes a Van Gogh red darkens to blue. Her arms and shoulders turn pallid. Below, on the river, the tide is rushing and tugboats push a flat barge upstream, and beyond that you can see the motionless dark skyline of midtown. At 5:00 or 6:00 A.M., when it was about to happen, a nurse came and woke you. You stood, tightening the drawstring of your greens, stuffed bare feet into your shoes, and came down the hall. It was quiet. The clerk was nodding off, and the smell of coffee the nurses were brewing filled the air. As you entered the sky shown through the window with that peculiar luminescence of New York dawn, a liquidity of hydrocarbons and sulfur and the humid exhalations of fifteen million lungs.

When you are certain, you pull your hand away. There are things to do.

The ritual is as old as a consciousness of death. Shamans or Egyptian embalmers may have been the first to distinguish with certainty between living and dead, but now it's the intern's job. You cover the floor while everyone else sleeps; you must wake the son in Teaneck or Brooklyn and tell him. Not much is worse than calling a man you've never met to tell him his mother has died. The groan. The long, half-awake silence. The oh, no. The oh, what should I do now? Should I come in? I should come in, shouldn't I? And then, when it no longer matters, everything is rushed and curiously urgent. You call the private doc, you fill out forms with time and circumstances of death, the clerk phones the information desk, nurses prepare the body for the family. Then they're in, dazed, unevenly shaven, drowsy-eyed, and in need of coffee. When they see you and hear your voice, pain comes to their faces, for in telling them, you brought it on. Now you'll hurt them again. When you ask them to give consent for an autopsy — a postmortem examination or a "post" — the fact of death slices into them. Why do you have to do that? they ask. No, don't, please don't. It's over; she suffered enough.

Sometimes you don't fight them, but at other times you feel compelled to. For weeks you may have been trying to find out what was killing the woman and all the tests came back negative, and the fever continued even though you used all the right antibiotics and tapped every cavity for fluid, and the heart resolutely failed despite the latest drugs. You need to know why. You have to fight them for it then, sometimes underhandedly. On the plains of Ilion, outside Troy, the Achaeans and the Trojans fought over the bodies of dead warriors, an invisible battle that raged and still rages to determine who'll recover the corpse for the end they think best. That battle is yours and theirs, and to either side loss is a kind of degradation. The comparison to Homer, you know, is not extreme.

"Now comes the real question," said our chief resident. "How do you get the post?"

It was noontime in July, a few days after internship had started, and we, the new interns, had been called down to the Medicine Library for lunch. Through the chief's introductory remarks about the importance of the autopsy in the progress of medical science, we ate sandwiches and drank Cokes and dozed and looked out dusty windows at the inaccessible sky. The chief introduced his buddy Jerry, one of the other residents. He was stocky, with a mustache, in rumpled whites. Now we woke. What we needed was not history but this, nuts and bolts. After all, we were the ones who, at 3:00 A.M., had to ask for a signature on a consent-to-autopsy form, and we were the ones blamed for failure on rounds the next morning. You didn't get the post on Mrs. Jacobs? We wanted it, you know.

"Number one," said Jerry, "when you ask the family for the post, don't reason with them. It's a waste of time. If you talk about the progress of science they'll walk out the door. Instead, listen to what they're saying. Whatever it is, agree one hundred percent. They always say one thing: 'He's suffered enough.' If you're rational, you'll say, 'What, are you crazy? He's dead. How the hell's an autopsy going to make him suffer anymore?' And they'll walk out the door. Instead, say, 'He did suffer enough. You're right. And I'll make sure he won't suffer anymore.' "

One of us interns had a question. "Just how do you keep the dead guy from suffering? Don't they ask that?"

He shook his head. "Never. Besides, I don't give them time, because I'm ready with number two: 'I'll be there.' Not some pathologist down in the morgue, but *me*, the doc who took care of Mom or Dad when they were still alive. 'I'll be there.' Am I always there? Not always. I do check up on what they find. Sometimes I go by there, sometimes I just call up. It's important to them, though, to *think* of me there, so I say it.

"Number three," he said. "The cutting. Don't go into detail. They don't want to hear about the brain sliced up and the liver cut into little pieces. They want to hear that Dad or Mom's not going to be mutilated. So tell them, 'It's just a small surgical procedure.' "

The overriding principle, it seemed, was to tell them whatever they wanted to hear. We stirred, disturbed by his recommendations. He disposed of religious objections — "There aren't any. We have an Orthodox rabbi who'll come in to watch; we have a priest and a minister who'll talk to the family." He told us how to get consent from relatives in another state. We flipped through the stapled handout he had given us: "Principle I: Sincerity; Principle II: Understanding Human Defenses During Period Immediately Following Death." We whispered among ourselves. Our skepticism may have come from the scientific cast of our minds, and our discomfort was perhaps a result of the ethic of informed consent, in which risks and complications are plainly explained. Maybe we just didn't feel comfortable being manipulative.

"Now this year," said the chief, "like last year, the Department of Medicine is giving prizes. Most autopsies obtained, most complete autopsies, highest percentage of patients receiving autopsies. We'll have prizes in all categories. As many as possible."

At that point we nudged one another in amazement. We laughed aloud. No one could believe prizes.

"Is there a prize for the intern with the least number of deaths?" one of us asked.

"That's what you get paid for," said the chief.

*

In his intellectual history of medicine, *The Birth of the Clinic*, Michel Foucault discusses the popular conception that early anatomists, among them Valsalva and Morgagni, were persecuted for performing autopsies. For one hundred and fifty years, Foucault says, it was generally believed that the opposition of organized religion, morality and emotional prejudice made autopsies dangerous and illegal. Supposedly, Valsalva could pursue his studies only by sneaking into graveyards, and Morgagni by digging up the graves of the dead and taking corpses from their coffins.

"This reconstitution," says Foucault, "is historically false." In eighteenth-century France autopsies were performed without interference by church or state. Yet historians of medicine have distorted what actually happened, creating opposition where none existed. Why did this distortion occur? Perhaps it is partly because the thought of the autopsy remains so disturbing to us. It is hard to keep our sense in dealing with a way of seeking the truth of life that proceeds through its destruction.

My first opportunity to test Jerry's advice came when Chiapas died. Simon Chiapas was a saturnine old Indian from Chile, with bristling white hair and a disease that puzzled everyone. Rashes, weight loss, shakes, fever, pains that came and went — all these tormented him. Fifty years he had lived in Brooklyn, after leaving Chile, but somehow he never learned English. So his wife had to translate his suffering to us. She was a short, gaudy Puerto Rican with hennaed hair, charm bracelets, and a habit of grabbing your white coat when she talked. Did Chiapas hurt anywhere? She translated, holding firm to your coat sleeve; he nodded or frowned. Where did he hurt? Shrug. His chest? Nod. His stomach? Nod. Which pain was the worst? Shrug. When I stuck a needle into his arm he screamed like a baby.

At morning rounds Mrs. Chiapas sat by his bedside with a

Spanish newspaper; in the afternoons she'd be there, licking the tip of her pencil to help her with her book of crossword puzzles. She wanted to know everything about the treatment. What disease did we think he had? How come he had those terrible high fevers? And his weight — why didn't he eat? Why was he getting so thin? Every day she asked the same questions, as if the coming of a new day erased the answers of the one before. And every day I answered again. We weren't sure what her husband had. Maybe tuberculosis, but none of the cultures had grown. Maybe an early form of leukemia, but then why was the bone marrow normal? Maybe lymphoma, but then we would have expected something abnormal on the CT scan. Maybe some rare disease from South America — after all, hadn't he gone back to Chile for a visit in the spring?

"The hematologist wants to do another bone marrow," I would announce. Or, "We're going to order some more X rays today." Or, "The Infectious Disease consultant says we should do another spinal tap." Mrs. Chiapas would groan, blot her eyes with a wad of tissues, and then translate to her husband, who lay still on the bed, wasted hands at his sides and eyelids heavy.

"Tell him it won't hurt very much."

She translated.

"We think it's really important." And again.

Five or ten minutes might elapse before Chiapas nodded.

"He will have it," she said.

Afterward she would follow me out in the hall and grab me by the sleeve of my coat.

"Tell me, Doctor, between you and me, what do you think it is?"

I would explain yet again.

"But why? Why does this happen?"

"Mrs. Chiapas, I'm very sorry, but we're doing our best."

"I know, I know you are." Then she wept. "But the tests hurt him so much. And what do you find? Nothing."

Then, one day when I came to get consent for another study — I forget which one — she crumpled her newspaper in her hands and shook her head back and forth.

"It doesn't hurt."

"I don't want him tortured no more."

There was no way to argue with her. Anyway, we were at a standstill. High-dose steroids had only puffed him up with an unnatural bloated shine, four antibiotics were at work wrecking his kidneys, and even with Tylenol every few hours he had fevers of a hundred and five. Next I would be injecting an antifungal agent into his spinal canal every day. I knew that would be torture.

So we delayed. She wanted to think about it; I didn't hurry her. Then he died. The family watched me closely during the final hours, as I came in to turn the IV faster or slower, or to inject drugs or peer at his dilated, unmoving pupils. Mrs. Chiapas was there and an old Indian with black glasses and a thin young man I hadn't seen before, and they watched my every move. Me, the torturer. Finally there was nothing. I pulled my stethoscope away and nodded. They all went hysterical with grief. Mrs. Chiapas fell against the young man's shoulder; the old Indian started shouting.

I left to fill out the papers. Time of death was 3:27 P.M. Witnesses were one of the nurses and me. Cause of death I left blank. Consent to autopsy was next. I dreaded asking for it, but there was no choice. So I went to get her.

She came out into the hallway, moaning and bumping into things. When I asked her to sign, it was just as Jerry had said.

"No, Doctor, he suffered enough already."

I was ready with what Jerry had recommended. "I know. He *has* suffered enough."

Her red eyes stared me down. "Listen, Doctor, I ain't going

to let you cut him up, understand? You tortured him long enough when he was alive, understand?"

"I . . . I'll make sure he won't suffer anymore."

"How?" she said. "How you going to make sure? You been lying to me all along, now you just make more lies to me. I ain't signing nothing."

A long pause ensued. This had not been part of Jerry's scenario.

"Can I ask why you don't want it?"

"Because I don't want him all cut up, understand? And you won't find out nothing. When he was alive you didn't find out nothing, so what for should I let you cut him up now?"

I left her to the young man and the old Indian, and went to the nurses' station to finish my paperwork. What killed Chiapas was less to her than that he was dead. But I wanted to know. And more, I wasn't going to let her win. In the space for listing cause of death, I wrote *unknown*.

Soon the information desk called me.

"You can't write *unknown* as the cause of death," the clerk said.

"It *is* *unknown*. We have no idea why he died."

"That's going to make it a coroner's case, Doctor."

"Whatever the rules are," I said.

An hour later, someone telephoned from the office of the chief medical examiner of New York City. It was a young-voiced woman, probably just out of residency training.

"You have a Simon Chiapas?"

"Sure do," I said. "A great case." I told her about the weight loss, fevers, diarrhea, the lingering and mysterious decline. I felt compelled to sell her the case, to make it intriguing, more mysterious than it was. Not exactly lying, just presenting it in a way I thought might appeal to a coroner. "One thing we considered," I said, "was the possibility of infection. This guy went back to Chile recently —"

"When was that?"

"Oh, two, three months ago," I said. "We were wondering about some rare South American parasite or a fungus. Maybe something contagious."

"Could be," said the pathologist. She paused a moment, reflecting. "We'll take him."

I went to explain to Mrs. Chiapas. The nurses had pulled the curtain around Chiapas's bed and removed the IVs and washed off the body and put clean sheets on the bed. Chiapas looked good. Mrs. Chiapas, her reddened eyes squeezed shut, was huddled in a chair, and she didn't open them when I told her about the medical examiner. She rocked from side to side.

"Why? Why do you got to do this to him? Please don't do it."

"The coroner," I said.

"I ain't going to let them cut him up."

"I don't know if you have any choice," I said. I left her there, by him, crying. I felt terrible.

As I was about to leave for the day, I was paged down to the information desk in the front lobby. The clerk handed me typed forms to sign.

"What took you?" he asked. "The undertaker's been waiting for an hour."

I looked around the lobby at patients in wheelchairs, policemen, visitors coming in the revolving doors.

"I don't understand. This was supposed to be a coroner's case."

"Well, it isn't. Maybe the family didn't want it. See, usually they don't fight the family."

"So what do I put as the cause of death, since we don't know?"

"Now you can put down *unknown*, since the medical examiner cleared it."

"Oh," I said. I put down *unknown*.

On rounds the next morning, another resident asked what had happened. I explained how none of Jerry's techniques had made any difference. He shook his head; it was one of the minor disappointments of the day.

"Too bad. We wanted it, you know." Then he grinned. "Did you try the gold ball story?"

"What's that?"

"You tell the family that just before the patient died you had him swallow a gold ball for a test and now it's stuck inside. The gold ball is worth five thousand dollars, and if you don't do the autopsy it's added to the hospital bill."

"That's sick," I said. "Who would say that?"

"Well, did you get the post?"

"No, the damn coroner gave in."

"They always do," he said. "They won't fight the family. It's up to you to get it."

"I know," I said. "Next time I will."

In Homer's *Iliad*, the rituals of death and after death are no less exact. Warriors fall, their bodies are stripped of armor, time after time the tide of battle turns around the recovery of a corpse. If won, it can be properly buried; if lost, it is open to desecration. After the Trojan hero Hector dies, stabbed through the neck by Achilles, his body is taken back to the Achaeans' camp. Achilles drags the dead Hector behind his chariot and sets dogs on him, and Achaean warriors stab him with their spears. But the gods protect Hector, who remains miraculously pure, unharmed. On the battlefield, the fighting has turned decisively in favor of the Achaeans. It is only a matter of time before Troy is taken; what causes more grief in Troy than impending defeat, however, is the thought of what is happening to Hector's corpse. So Hector's father,

Priam, goes before Achilles to bargain for the body. He appeals to him as a son whose own father lives in misery and affliction — can he not understand the grief of a father who has lost his sons? And Achilles, who, as Apollo says, "has destroyed pity," who, like a lion, has "gone among the flocks of men, to devour them," is moved to tears. In his one act of mercy in what has been an orgy of murder, he allows Priam to drive the body of Hector back to Troy, and promises to hold off attacking until Hector can be properly burned and mourned. For nine days, the men of Troy bring timber into the city and make a pyre on which to burn Hector's corpse. Hector is burned; then the pyre is doused with wine, and the white bones of Hector are gathered into a golden casket and buried. A "glorious feast" is held. Then the Trojans are freed to await their own destruction with equanimity.

The next post I really cared about was Zabell's. Morton Herbert Zabell was a furrier from Queens whose life was nothing extraordinary — he had married, fathered two children, managed a small business — until he got sick. Then he was swept from hospital to hospital, from specialist to a superspecialist, a large-boned man with a gloomy face, compiling charts and X-ray folders full of puzzling results. Finally he was sent to the Neurology Service of my hospital, nearly dead. I was on Neurology then, and six months of sleepless nights had made me more than a little Machiavellian. We revived him with steroids and repeated every test that had been done elsewhere, hoping for answers. We liked him. Nurses would come by and hold his hand and talk, and we interns were attentive to small comforts surrounding blood drawing and the placement of IV lines.

His dying was appalling and remarkable. Not only was it slow, it happened every day. He had developed a rare fungal meningitis, which caused swelling of the passages draining spinal fluid from around the brain. Every so often the ICU nurse would come by to tell me Zabell's pupils were getting big.

"They've blown again?"

"The left is five millimeters, the right seven. And they don't react."

"Is the mannitol ready?" I asked, hurrying toward his room. Zabell lay in bed, the pupils large black holes in his head, his arms and legs rigid, occasionally twitching. I grabbed a fifty-cc syringe and began pushing mannitol solution. When the syringe was empty, I pushed another and another. Then we waited.

"They're shrinking down," the nurse said.

"Give me a light." I shone it into his eyes. The pupils twitched and seemed to narrow for a fraction of a second. "I think they're reacting."

He would pop out of it. He would move his arms and legs, look at us, perhaps say a thing or two. Mrs. Zabell would come back into the room, moaning, praising us, squeezing his bloated hand. She was frail and harried, and try as I might I couldn't calm her fears.

"Is he okay, Doctor? Tell me he's okay, huh?"

This was a daily occurrence with Zabell, and eventually we came to accept this miraculous recovery from what is called herniation as commonplace. Mrs. Zabell refused to understand how serious things were. She had fewer questions than Mrs. Chiapas, but more theories.

"Do you think he caught it from the pigeons? Huh?" she asked. "There's an overpass near our house, and a lot of pigeons live under the bridge. Do you think he could have caught it from them?"

She had hypotheses about the dogs, too, from whom Zabell

had once caught worms. She remembered the box turtle that one of the children had brought home from elementary school years ago. She wondered if she herself might have given it to him; she wasn't so sure about her cooking. She advanced her desperate guesses in the hallways, she interrupted rounds with queries, she found me by the elevators to wonder if it was something in the pastrami. She begged me to allow her to spend the night.

"Please, Doctor, I'll just stay in the chair. Or I'll sleep in the lounge. I won't make a word, I won't bother a thing. I can't go home to Queens now. Morton needs me."

In the middle of the night she had me awakened by the nurses.

"Do you think I can go home now? I just remembered, Doctor, I have to feed the dogs. Please, Doctor, say I can leave . . ."

No one, including me, could figure out what to do with her. She was so foolish and so sad that one couldn't get angry at her. And I had an idea what was coming. Each time Zabell herniated, something was lost. It is as Foucault says, paraphrasing the eighteenth-century French anatomist Bichat:

> Death is therefore multiple, and dispersed in time; it is not that absolute, privileged point at which time stops and moves back; like disease itself, it has a teeming presence that analysis may divide into time and space; gradually, here and there, each of the knots breaks until organic life ceases, at least in its major forms, since long after the death of the individual, minuscule, partial deaths continue to disassociate the islets of life that still subsist.

One time Zabell blew his pupils, and the mannitol injections brought back only one side. On his left he was flaccid as a rag doll. For a few hours strength returned; then it departed for good. Then he lost sensation. To a needle jab or a

bruising pinch there was no response, not a twitch or a grimace. When our team was at X-ray rounds, he stopped
breathing; by the time we got back to the floor, Zabell was
on a respirator. The pupils blew, responded to mannitol, and
blew again. All four limbs were permanently paralyzed. He
lay with eyes half opened, like a pithed lab frog. Gas bloated
up his belly. A nauseating odor filled the room. How much
simpler, I couldn't help thinking, were the deaths of warriors
on the plains of Ilion.

When Zabell went, both children were there — a college-
student daughter and a bearded cab driver son in yellow, high-
top Keds and a sweater. I came in with my stethoscope to
confirm that he was dead. I listened, I felt for a pulse, I nodded. Mrs. Zabell fell on the bed so hard she almost knocked
the dead man out of it. The children had to grab her to keep
her from the other patients in the room.

I stood there until she was under control, then went to get
the forms. This time I wasn't going to fail. No matter what, I
would get that post. The mercy that moved Achilles wouldn't
have a ghost of a chance in me. I figured the best way to get
it was to use the children, use them against their mother. I
took the three of them out to the alcove by the elevators, the
only private place on the floor, and told them about the
autopsy.

"No, I don't want you to do it," said Mrs. Zabell. "He
suffered too much already."

"I know," I said. "I know this is a terrible time to ask. I
know he suffered enough." He suffered enough — it was not
so much a platitude as a basic human discovery. But I could
agree only in a tactical sense, while preparing to subvert. I
had an odd feeling then, which came and went in a matter of
seconds, and I didn't know what to think of it, the conviction
that I was leaving the human race.

Nodding gravely, I fixed my attention on the children.

"I think we want it," I said.

Moaning, Mrs. Zabell threw her weight against her daughter. I let her cry. Entirely unmoored, the cab driver stared at me. It hadn't hit him yet that his father was dead. I motioned him around the corner.

"If I were you," I said, "if it was my father, I think I would want the autopsy. I'd want to *know.*"

He shook his head.

"This is it," I said. "This is your one chance to know. What if it's something hereditary? You may have the same disease. Or an infection. Maybe the whole family should be treated. Wouldn't you want to know?"

He leaned against the wall. I was getting to him.

"And look at your mother. She thinks it's her fault. Pigeons, dogs, the box turtle even. For the rest of her life she'll think it's her fault. If we can show her that it's not — say that it's cancer . . ."

He swallowed.

"It's up to you," I said.

"Okay. Let me talk to my sister."

When he took his sister aside, the old lady fell against me, crying. I stood there, holding her, while the two of them talked. I heard the elevators moving in their shafts, distantly rising and falling, stopping on other floors, moving past, and around the corner the son and daughter talking, deciding what to do.

They came back.

"We want it," said the taxi driver.

"She'll have to sign for it," I said.

"I'm going to sign for nothing," she said.

There was a wooden bench by the elevator, and I led her there and sat her down and put the clipboard on her lap and a pen in her right hand.

"Sign right there," I said.

Her hand shook. "I don't want to hurt him." She cried.

"I'll be there," I said.

"Mom, you got to," said the son.

"Sign it," I said. I led her narrow hand to the paper and held it there until it began to write.

Next morning my resident and I went down to Pathology to check out Zabell. On my own I might not have gone, but my Neurology resident had a hotshot theory about the cause of death and was set to impress the professor. Besides, I *had* told the wife I'd be there. We approached Pathology through narrow corridors lined with shelves of specimens in jars and huge glass urns with organs in cloudy formalin. We came on a big central room where the gross dissection was done, and there lay Zabell in a big stainless steel sink, naked, a long Y-shaped incision in his belly, and the top of his skull was sawed off and lay to the side like a beggar's bowl. On a little platform were his liver, heart and kidneys. A Pathology resident came over.

"We have only the gross specimens so far," he said. "Nothing remarkable. A little cirrhosis in the liver, an old myocardial infarction. Now, the brain's another matter. Swollen meninges. Looks like disseminated Cryptococcus."

"We already knew that," I said.

"Well, that's about it," he said.

"Did you find the gold ball?" I asked.

They both looked at me.

"What?"

"Nothing. Actually, we were interested in what underlying disease may have predisposed him to the Crypto."

The Pathology resident shrugged. "Come back in a few days."

"I will," I assured him.

I didn't go back. There were reasons: I was about to leave Neurology and was busy writing off-service notes on one ward and on-service notes on another; the holidays were close enough to set my mind on other things. And somehow it didn't seem crucial to find out — not to me, anyway. The neurologists could have a conference on it. I felt satisfied that I had won. It was like the bright, disturbing detail, which Homer recounts on the battlefield outside Troy as the fighting turns around the bodies of young dead soldiers. Even though the larger battle might be lost, the smaller defeats hurt more, and the small victories give a kind of consolation. I claimed Zabell for our knowledge, which was what really counted.

It was nearly the end of internship when I ran into my Neurology resident in the hospital elevator and remembered to ask about Zabell. My resident was dressed in shorts and a T-shirt and carried a squash racquet in his hand.

"Zabell?"

"You know," I said. "The guy with disseminated Crypto. What did the slides show?"

"Oh, him. He was a real surprise. Lung cancer with brain mets."

"Lung cancer? You're kidding."

"Nope. Never would have suspected it when he was alive. We thought it was a T-cell defect, something exotic. They found the goobers in his head first — metastatic adenocarcinoma. And they had to look all over to find a primary. It was a coin lesion in the right lung."

"How come the CT scan didn't show it?"

"I don't know. Maybe he moved around, maybe the resolution wasn't good. I think they used the old machine with him."

"It's incredible," I said.

"Yeah. Makes you feel better. Nothing we could have done, anyhow. Lucky we got the post, huh?"

We were on my floor then. I held the door open with my hand for a moment and looked at him in his gym shorts.

"*I* got it," I said. Then the door closed and he went on up toward the squash courts and I went back to my patients. I did get it; that was what counted, after all. What else was won or lost should be a matter of indifference to me.

The Madonna of
Red Hook

WHEN MY AUNT MIMI heard what I wanted to be she begged me not to do it. The whole family was at her house in Shaker Heights for Uncle Ed's birthday. I was in my last year of medical school and had stopped in town on my way East for residency interviews. Aunt Mimi grabbed my arm. Aunt Mimi squeezed. Chocolate layer cake and Neapolitan ice cream nearly spilled from my paper plate onto wall-to-wall carpet.

"Don't do it!" she said. "It's a terrible business!"

"What do you mean?" I said.

"They're . . . they're a bunch of quacks. And worse. Why don't you do something real, like your father?"

All around us chubby cousins and gray uncles were eating chocolate layer cake and Neapolitan ice cream. I sipped Hawaiian Punch. I tried to think of a way to explain how intensely bored I was by internal medicine, my father's field, and how psychiatry seemed to offer so much more — more what I didn't exactly know — but Aunt Mimi had already turned to my little sister, to find how basketball practice was going, and my answer was forgotten.

The question, however, was repeated a number of times in the next few months. My endocrinology fellow tormented me with it. "I hear you're planning to throw away your medical education," he said. And when in one consultation I suggested that the patient see a psychiatrist, he insisted that I remove my note from the chart and write a new one.

And that December, after I finished the Psychiatry residency application process and was waiting to be accepted, I was accosted at a party by a stooped, vaguely clerical man who said he was a psychiatrist — a psychoanalyst.

"I hear you want to be a psychiatrist," he said. "Well, if you're looking for a quiet, comfortable life, don't do it. Forget it. Do something else." He looked at me gloomily. "Why do you want to do it?"

But before I could answer, the evening was over.

I spent that winter trying to make up my mind. Was I going to follow my father into internal medicine, which required sacrifice and dedication? Or was I going to veer into the thickets of psychiatry, and spend all my time with crazies?

Two years later, there I was, a Psychiatry resident, sitting in conference with other Psychiatry residents and medical students and social workers and nurses and our professor, Dr. Valtin, listening to the presentation of a new patient and wondering why the decision had been so quick, whether it was only the reaction of an oppositional nature, or if there was more to it.

My medical student Ellen was presenting. She was curly haired and enthusiastic about seeing as many patients as she could. She was applying to my program, and every time she spoke I was tempted to shout at her, "Don't do it!"

"Mrs. Racusi is a twenty-one-year-old married waitress who delivered a baby son by caesarian section three days prior to admission, and who became psychotic the next day. She has no previous psychiatric history. After she was brought home she became agitated and put her arm through a window . . ."

Mrs. Racusi's madness was a Brooklyn madness, a low-voltage affair of scrambled thoughts and mutterings and halfhearted impulses to suicide, all flavored with paranoia. It was not one of those electrifying, soul-shaking, wrist-slashing, overdosing Manhattan insanities, which threaten spontaneous combustion of the crazy one and dozens of innocent bystanders and could snarl traffic for hours. Mrs. Racusi would not even have come to our unit, in fact, if not for the accident of a window coming between her fist and the phantom face of her sister-in-law Donna Marie.

So I sat back as Ellen talked, wondering if Aunt Mimi was right. Perhaps there was more to her warning than I had realized; perhaps the fate of sitting in a room listening to a flood of misery and pain was a terrible one for a boy from Cleveland Heights; perhaps I should have figured this out before making my choice of residency, a choice for life. One thing was becoming apparent after some months of inpatient psychiatry — that our planet was overrun with craziness and anguish (at least in the vicinity of Manhattan), that the world's only unlimited resource was human pain. Not only that, but to sit immobile for hour after hour, listening, was to be blamed for what the world had inflicted, to have your very soul scorched. And to be reminded time after time how much could not be done.

They brought her into conference mad. She was mumbling to the walls, a shuffling woman with ashen Mediterranean skin and hair black and glittery as coal, bodiless and tangled, and a belly still so big that her shirt rode up over it and she had not been able to snap her jeans shut. Her face, a dark Madonna's round face, was void of tenderness.

"Sit down, Mrs. Racusi," said Dr. Valtin.

She stared at Valtin a moment, sat gingerly, surveyed us in horror, stood, began to talk, sat down, reached for the bandage on her arm, picked idly, said the name Donna Marie, asked if any of us had a joint.

"I've heard a little about you," said Dr. Valtin. "But perhaps you could tell us in your own words . . ."

Awed, she watched him, as if bugs were crawling from his mouth. She giggled. Clearly she was undermedicated, this Madonna from Red Hook, Brooklyn, waitress on maternity leave, madwoman. Poor grooming, inappropriate affect, hallucinations; an embarrassment to the unit, a disturbance to other patients. Well, anyway, in a few weeks we'd have her saturated with medications and back to her apartment.

"I saw Donna Marie in the window, I wanted to punch her, she wants to take my baby away, she's my husband's sister and she thinks she can take my baby . . . and I want my baby back because she's going to drown him in the bathtub and then she'll laugh . . . I heard her say she was going to do it . . . can I leave? I don't want to talk about it anymore, I just want to go home . . . Why can't I go home?"

"Where's the baby?" asked Dr. Valtin after she left.

"At the sister-in-law's."

"It's all right?"

Ellen nodded.

"This is the biggest problem in postpartum reactions," said Dr. Valtin. "Infanticide. There's a very high risk. People don't want to hear about it, but it's real, it happens." He sighed. "It's true these psychotic reactions are not usually schizophrenic in origin, that they're usually from an underlying manic-depressive illness. But they're much more difficult to treat. It's often a year or more before they resolve. What have you got her on?"

"Lithium and Prolixin."

"I would certainly go up on the antipsychotic medicine," said Dr. Valtin.

After conference, Ellen walked down the hall with me.

"It's really interesting," she said, "don't you think? I'm having the whole family come in today, so I can find out what really happened with Donna Marie."

"That's fine," I said. "But, like Valtin said, she needs more meds."

I went to my office, which was on the unit, between the rooms of two patients. After four months here I still had nothing on the walls, and only a few books. My desk was covered, though, with memos, forms to fill out, stacks of Xeroxed articles, including a manila folder from Dr. Valtin — the literature on postpartum reactions, biologic and analytic. I paged through it. What could it tell me about this woman, a waitress, high school graduate, wife, a decent, unexceptional woman? Why was she here? And why so sick? What was it about childbirth that made the illness so much worse? I read. The analysts had something to say, psychobiologists a little more. But none could provide answers, none seemed to do much other than hint at solutions; then they became cloudy, formulaic. To step beyond the visible seemed to lead nowhere. There were no unruly clones of cells, no viruses, no miscoded proteins in psychiatry as there were in medicine, no magic-bullet antibiotics, no radically corrective surgeries — not yet, anyway — and it seemed there was no likelihood of any being found for a long time. Instead, there was only silence, and understanding, some faint grasp of the anatomy of misery, and a few palliative drugs.

Someone next door was banging on a wall. I looked around. The walls were all yellowed by tobacco smoke, and on one side hung a green metal cabinet, left from the days when medications were kept here. The room seemed to be filled with

the reverberations of strange voices, recountings of precipi-
tous declines, the reliving of protracted family quarrels, con-
fessions of odd and impulsive acts, the residue of discarded
rationalizations. The time spent here — listening, dictating,
dialing the phone to reach psychiatrists in their country
houses, patients' families in New Jersey and Queens — could
seem endless; the room could seem to have an existence
only in relation to madness and to nothing else; there could
seem to be nothing outside.

The curtain on the door was pulled aside; someone was
looking in. I went to the door.

"Doctor? Is this the right day to see you?" It was Mrs.
Greenstone, who was getting shock treatments for depression
and was confused.

"No, tomorrow," I said.

"Oh, oh, I'm sorry, Doctor. What day is it?"

I told her; she wandered off down the hall.

Bill was my next appointment. A corporate lawyer at a
midtown firm, he had met a beautiful, deranged woman at a
bad time in his life, and overdosed when she got tired of him.
He was blond, heavyset as a plumber, and he hated and feared
doctors of all kinds.

"When are you going to let me out of this damn place?" he
said. He leaned forward in his chair. "You shrinks are real
sons of bitches, you know that?"

Bill was treated with antidepressants and psychotherapy over
the next month, and pretty soon he was well enough to go
back to his contracts. Ellen left, too, after a six-week rotation
on the unit, undiminished in her enthusiasm for finding out
everything about her patients, but unfortunately not for writing it in the charts. Mrs. Greenstone responded excellently to
electroconvulsive therapy, got the better part of her memory

back, and returned to Riverdale. But Mrs. Racusi stayed.

The trees in the courtyard in front of the hospital lost their leaves, and the ground became packed by rain. Behind the building the river was as discolored as an old pipe. The unit filled with people for whom Thanksgiving had been too much, and the approach of Christmas and the new year brought thoughts of jumping and slashing. I silver-taped my window to stop the draft from killing my plants.

Mrs. Racusi spent her days in bed. I'd write an appointment time on the bulletin board and wait in my office for her to come in. But most of the time I'd have to walk all the way around the floor to her room, knock on the door, and go in, to find her lying in bed, fully dressed and asleep.

"Come on, it's time to meet."

"Oh, I'm sorry, Doctor," she'd say. "I'll be there."

I'd walk the long corridor back to my office and wait. Finally she would arrive, with bright splotches of lipstick smeared over her mouth and eyeshadow making coal smudges of her eyes.

"So what's up?"

"I want to go home to Red Hook. I want to see my baby."

"We'll have him come here," I said. "Soon."

"I don't want to see him *here*, not with all these crazy people."

"That's the way we have to do it."

She giggled.

I asked what it was.

"I want a joint. Do you think if I gave you five dollars you could get me a joint? I'd do anything to have some Thai stick." She rambled on. Out the window I could see the gray tower of the main hospital, the bare tops of trees, cabs lined up to get back to the avenue. Mrs. Racusi was better than when she had come in, but not much. If we cut the Prolixin back too much she became crazy again; if we increased the dose, she spent the whole day in bed. And as far as I could tell the Lithium wasn't doing a damn thing. How much easier it was in the main hospital, where you drew blood and scheduled X rays and didn't have to listen. On Obstetrics it had been even better. The big-bellied women came in dilated, contracting. They'd walk up and down the corridors in their bathrobes and slippers, trying to convince gravity to do the work of time; nothing would happen. You'd wait forever; you and the resident would go to bed on cots in rumbling, shaking internal rooms, and hours would pass, until suddenly you'd be awakened by the nurses and run down the tiled halls to find everything ready, the waters broken, sometimes the head crowning out, and you'd guide what nature began, finding a gray-blue warm creature that seemed drowned, entirely dead, but would start moving, shudder, breathe, and in a few minutes be pink, crying, alive, being wrapped in a blanket off to the side as you remembered to pull the veiny cord so the placenta, like some strange sea fruit, splashed into a metal pan. Then you'd clamp and cut the cord, and the wrapped baby would be laid on the mother's breast, and it would be as if you'd accomplished something extraordinary, and of course you had. But this. Here the waiting produced no miraculous existence, no transfiguration, no event.

"When can I go home?" she asked.

"When do you think?"

They brought the baby in, by car service from Brooklyn, on a snowy day. Dr. Valtin insisted that everything be arranged in advance, so she would be observed at all times, not disturbed by other patients, and so the visit would not last too long. Her husband, Sal, and his worried sister, Donna Marie, both Northern Italian blonds, were in the room when I came by, standing over the bed. The baby lay there on his back. He was pink, gurgling, dressed in a snowsuit. Donna Marie was doing something right. Way over by the window, her back to everyone, arms limp at her sides, stood Mrs. Racusi.

"She don't want to touch him, Doctor," said Sal. "She played with him for a minute and that was it. Now she says take him back to Brooklyn."

"How come?"

"She says —"

"I don't want him!" she said. "Donna Marie wants him, she can keep him. So take him away, okay? I don't want him."

They took him away, but the next day she said she wanted him back. This time she held him stiffly on her thigh, all the way down at her knee, and looked off into space as she fed him. She held the bottle on the level rather than above his head, so mostly he swallowed air. The nurse would tilt the bottle up, but if you came back a few minutes later there it would be, level again.

But she pulled it together. Not as fast as most people — most people are ready to go in less than a month — but fast enough. She got it into her mind that she wanted to be out for the holidays, so if there was any way to speed things up . . .

We got a crib from Pediatrics, a big thing with black rubber wheels and metal-barred sides that slid up and down, and the baby began to spend the night. The nurses checked up on them a few times an hour. She began holding him better, talking to him, changing diapers. Everyone was impressed with how much she'd improved.

"So what's the plan?" Dr. Valtin asked one afternoon.

"We're going to discharge her in about a week. She'll have the baby, she'll be going to the day hospital, she'll continue her medication . . ."

"Has she said anything about hurting the baby?"

Battles of Life and Death

"No."

"Even any suggestion? Anything that would indicate she was defending against impulses to —"

"No!" I was annoyed. Why did Dr. Valtin always harp on that same issue? Faulty mothering and murderous wishes and secret infanticide — didn't we get the idea already? If you could give a pill for murderous wishes, fine.

"Well, all we can do is worry."

When the family came — a week before Christmas — we filled the river lounge with chairs. All the Racusis were there — Sal in his silver leather jacket, Donna Marie in a fur coat, with the baby on her hip, two pudgy brothers, old Mrs. Racusi, who was all grays and blacks. *Her* family, the Altanos, were there too — her mother, her elderly stepfather, her brother Danny and his wife. Mrs. Racusi sat in an armchair, looking at the floor.

"Well, let's start," said Jeanne, the social worker.

"I got something to say," said Danny Altano.

"Can you wait a few minutes? I want to make sure that everyone's —"

"No, I ain't going to wait. What I want to know is how come Donna Marie's been doing all this shit with the baby. I mean, my sister's been right all along. Donna Marie *does* want to take that baby for herself, and she's doing everything she can to keep it."

"That's bullshit," said Donna Marie.

"No it isn't," said Danny's wife.

"Yes it is," said Donna Marie. "I been staying up all night taking care of that baby and now she's going to get it back. I'm *still* willing to help with the baby if she needs help, and I haven't seen you around once, and I don't care if you live in Fort Lee, you could still do something."

"We are going to do something. When she don't want the

baby, when she wants a rest, *we'll* take the baby, okay? We don't want your help anymore, okay?"

"Oh yeah? Where you been? Where you been all these months?"

Then they all started in. It was the Racusis against the Altanos at first, then it was Mrs. Altano against her son Danny, and then Donna Marie started shouting at *her* mother, and the two pudgy brothers started complaining, and Sal Racusi walked out of the room and had to be brought back by Donna Marie, and the two of them stood outside the room jabbing at each other, and all the other ones stood in a group, yelling at Jeanne and me, and Jeanne and I said everything we could think of to bring some order and shut up when the screaming continued anyway. Then I just watched Mrs. Racusi, dark, plump in her sack dress, the baby now flopped over her, face in her breast, and behind everything, out the dusty windows, the icy rolling river and, above, the gray cumulus atmosphere of winter.

"We're going to sign her out of the hospital right now!" Danny Altano screamed. "This fucking place only makes her sicker!"

She and the baby sat still.

A few days later she went home. They filled a bunch of cardboard boxes with her clothes and the baby's things and diapers and magazines and plastic bottles of lotion and get-well cards and baby cards, and they put the baby in a snowsuit and wrapped him in a blanket and Mrs. Racusi in a winter coat that scarcely buttoned over her belly, and they took her to the car service and drove her back to Red Hook. A schizophrenic got her room; the crib was moved out in the hall to be returned to Pediatrics, and somebody strung red and green crepe paper through its metal bars.

There was a long weekend for Christmas with a long weekend for New Year's coming up, and in the week between, everybody was angry. The aides tried to get out early; the nurses said no one ever listened to them; we residents complained that the administration had no idea what long hours we had to work; and overdosers and wrist slashers flooded the Emergency Room, trying to get into the hospital, which alone could save them from themselves. All the patients inside complained that we were keeping them against their will, that there was nothing wrong with them except the depressing atmosphere of the ward, and they threatened to sign out or run away. In short, things were going smoothly.

That Wednesday the head nurse paged me out of Grand Rounds.

"You've got an admission," she said.

"What do you mean? I'm not up."

"It's your little friend."

"My friend?"

"Racusi."

"You're kidding. What happened?"

"Oh, she stopped taking her meds — her husband didn't think she needed them. Then he had a Christmas party for her and she got stoned and started acting a little funny, and the next thing you know they found her out on the fire escape with the baby."

"Oh, no," I said.

"You sound so surprised," she said.

"I'm going to kill Donna Marie. Stick an icepick in her face. And twist it around. Hello, Doctor," said Mrs. Racusi when I came in. She smiled flirtatiously. "Do I have to stay here? I want to return my Christmas presents, I have a little sweater for my baby that's already too small. You know, he was ten pounds when he was born. Why do I have to be here? I want my old room back. I went there and there's somebody else in my room —"

"Why didn't you take your meds?"

"I did. Oh, I took everything, Doctor. And last night I had some wine and got stoned with my brother and his friends, a little New Year's present, and oh, I have a really good party to go to tonight in the Village. I wonder if it's going to snow —"

"What about the baby?"

"The baby?"

"On the fire escape. What were you doing out there?"

She laughed.

"Tell me."

"It was too crowded. I wanted some air —"

"I can't believe it," I said. You always sent patients out, knowing they wouldn't take their medications or go to their doctors, that they'd resume their most destructive habits. But Mrs. Racusi was different; she'd had a baby with her out there on the fire escape. I couldn't get the image out of my mind.

We began the medications again. We pushed the doses as high as she could tolerate, and still she was mumbling crazy things, trying to sneak into the elevators. Finally we gave up and began shock treatments, first a dozen, which made her better for a few weeks, then eight more when she started getting worse again. If you gave enough they were almost always supposed to work — enough shocks and you'd knock the craziness out of the brain, return the serotonin or dopamine, or whatever neurotransmitter was governing sanity, to its proper levels.

And it worked for her. It worked the way so much of medical treatment still works, interrupting disease but restoring something different from health. She was not crazy anymore,

but not right, either. There was a vacuity, an inaccessibility
of mind.

The baby began visiting again, and that brightened her up;
the rest of the day she might be in bed, but when the baby
was there, in his silver crib by the window, she'd stand by
him and smile and play. At first, when the baby was wrapped
up and taken back to Brooklyn, she'd begin getting blank again,
like an old television set whose picture shrinks and shrinks to
a bright dot, which gradually expires. But then she started
feeling better and would take passes to walk around in the
neighborhood, or call up her girlfriends at work and meet
them for lunch. She even went down to Brooklyn by subway
one day to meet her new doctor.

One Monday morning, on my way to rounds, I was surprised to see the crib out in the hall, by the water fountain.

"Mrs. Racusi went out on pass with her brother last night,"
said the nurse in report. "She was acting a little strange afterward."

Jeanne and I looked at each other.

"Strange how?"

"She doesn't want the baby to come today. She put the crib
out in the hall."

"I can't believe it," I said. Through the rest of report I sat
there miserably depressed. Here it was February, she'd been
here over four months, we'd been working like mad to help
her — and she had to blow it again. I knew what had happened last night with her brother; he'd gotten her stoned. That
alone was enough to set her loose again. I knew what I'd see
this morning. The same rambling, murderous talk, the same
idiocy about signing out of the hospital and Donna Marie
wanting the baby and the rest. Why bother? What stupidity
to spend all that effort time and again, to be compassionate,
patient, sincere, only to be brought to a standstill by the very

people you were trying to help. What was the point of it all?

Mrs. Racusi was worse than I expected. The babbling was as bad as it had been in October. We gave her more medication than ever before. But the baby crib began moving farther and farther down the hall — past the water fountain, around the corner, to the nurses' station and beyond, past the center lounge to the opposite corridor. And finally it stopped.

"Maybe we can't do anything more for her," Dr. Valtin said in conference one day. "We have to consider what our choices are."

"Like what?" I asked.

"We may have to transfer her to a state hospital. If they'll take her. Or we might have to send her home like this. And give the baby to someone else. There are some people we just can't help — we have to admit that."

I began thinking about my own alternatives. Perhaps it wasn't too late to apply to internal medicine programs — some of the other Psychiatry residents were talking about that. Or take a year off. And the women residents were talking about having babies.

With spring, Mrs. Racusi began getting better. Not a whole lot, but enough to relieve despair, for as the craziness left the depression came back, and the long days spent in bed, but she didn't talk about signing out or getting stoned with her brother; she wanted to get back to her baby and her husband. The crib rolled back to her room. The baby came in. And the family, too. Everyone talked like battlefield survivors. No one screamed; the Altanos and Racusis agreed to a plan where the baby would not come home, at least in the beginning. Donna Marie would keep him for the time being. No one had the energy to disagree.

And finally Mrs. Racusi left. We had set a deadline — the middle of the month — and when that day came she had to go whether or not she was ready. Otherwise there seemed to be no way to get her out.

The day she was to leave I met with her before rounds. She was waiting by my office door when I came in, which in itself seemed a good sign. Her makeup was more or less in the right locations on her face, she had brushed her dark hair, and she was wearing a big, loose, tentlike dress that made her look pregnant still — or again.

"I can't wait to get home," she said. She sat forward in the chair, talking about how she knew she shouldn't have another baby, about her medications and the day hospital and the way she felt better, even though it was hard to get out of bed in the mornings; still, her head was clear. Every so often there'd be a long pause — seconds, minutes, a timeless interval in which it seemed that the entire world must be in suspension and of which she would have no memory when it was over.

"What is it?" I said. And waited. The perimeters of silence seemed elastic, infinite, a blankness in which an entire confusing history could be repeated and forgotten.

"Nothing," she said.

"What?"

"I wasn't thinking," she said. "I was just waiting. You know, there are so many things I forget. Maybe it was the shock treatments, maybe sooner or later . . ."

"Yes?" I said when the pause had gotten too long.

"I don't know. Something." She looked me full in the face, smiling for a moment, then her gaze went to the window, outside of which the trees in the hospital courtyard were hazy with yellow-green, the beginnings of the idea of leaves. "What time is it, do you know? I wish I had my watch. I don't know where I put it. My husband's supposed to be here at nine."

The Electric Prince

WHEN I FIRST saw the prince he was doing his best to wrench his head off. With one hand on either side of his face, he was tugging and jerking and twisting, as though once he found the right position his head would suddenly disarticulate from his neck and end up in his hands. He seemed pretty sure what he'd do with it next, but oblivious to the impracticality of his methods. Jack and Eddie, the two male aides who were with him, were trying to loosen his hands from his cheeks.

I stood in the doorway with Kohlman.

"What do you mean, a prince?" I asked.

"He *is,*" Kohlman replied. Kohlman, one of my fellow residents, had been on call the night before, and he had the logy, unshaven look and the slurred voice of a man whose judgment may not be entirely reliable.

"Is what?" I said.

"A real prince. At first I thought it was a grandiose delusion — I had him pegged for a manic — but there were people from some estate in Jersey calling and a baroness drove him in. She'd been trying to manage him at home — doesn't believe in psychiatrists — but found him about to take all the pills in her medicine cabinet. So she called the . . ."

The prince was sixtyish, a bulky, unshaven man in a tweed jacket, which was torn in the armpits, and an untucked and none-too-clean white shirt, and he did a pretty good job of shaking off Jack and Eddie, who had to keep grabbing his forearms. Kohlman was saying something about the Emergency Room and neurologists and medical clearance.

"Why are you telling me this?" I said. I had drifted onto the unit only because shock treatments — June was my month to do them — had been delayed this morning, the anesthesiologist having been called to the main hospital for an emergency. I had passed Kohlman on the way to my office, and merely stopped to say hello.

"He's yours," Kohlman said. "You're up for a new patient, right?"

"Oh, *shit*," I answered. Then I woke up. "What's going on? He'll hurt himself. How come he's not in restraints?"

"He's a prince," Kohlman said.

"So?" I said. Kohlman had the habit, I had learned after a year on a psychiatric floor with him, of preferring philosophy over action, of reveling in observation and ethical musings. He could always find reason to delay. On the other hand, of course, Kohlman probably had as complete a catalogue of my deficiencies as I did of his.

"I suppose you're right," he said. "He's been doing this most of the night."

"How about some medication?"

"He refuses."

"What do you say we get some aides and a nurse with IM Haldol and a camisole and see what we can do," I suggested. Kohlman was wobbling. "Did you sleep?"

"No . . . three admissions . . . a heart failure on Three . . ."

I went for the nurses' station, leaving him behind.

Within ten minutes we had the prince in a brand-new, white canvas, brass-buckled camisole, with his arms crossed over his chest and connected to the bed frame by rolled bed sheets and adhesive tape. Even after a hefty shot of antipsychotics the prince was doing his best to flip over the bed. But things were under control. The extra aides had dispersed, the nurse had gone back to her station, and the only one left was Eddie, in a chair, with a copy of *Glamour* on his lap.

"So what is he — agitated depression?" I said.

"I think so," Kohlman said.

"And the treatment plan? We going to shock him?"

"Oh," said Kohlman, "I tried to talk them into it last night — the baroness and the other people. They won't even *listen* to the idea. They think he should have analysis."

"Analysis?"

"Yeah, analysis," he said. "But they'll be back this afternoon."

"Great," I said. "I always did well with royalty."

"So how many do we have today?"

I was the last one to the electroconvulsive therapy (ECT) suite that morning — the head nurse had tangled me up in rounds over the issue of whether Miss Cutler, my borderline, could handle an unaccompanied pass to Bloomingdale's, or whether she would just come back with razor blades again. By the time I arrived, the ECT nurse had gotten the first patient on the table, and the anesthesiologist, Dr. Rickey, in his crumpled whites, was growling over his suitcase of vials, tubes, syringes, airways and face masks, aggressively squirting poisonous drugs in my general direction on the pretext of getting air bubbles out of his syringes.

"Six," said the ECT nurse. Rickey and I always called her

ECT Mary because that was how she answered the phone. "Mrs. English ate graham crackers again."

"Too bad," I said. "She needs those treatments. Hello, Mrs. Goldman."

"Hello, Doctor." Mrs. Goldman, the woman on the table, was wrinkled and arthritic, with a big square forehead on which it was easy to get the electrodes to stay. Before we began the treatments she had decided all water was "poison ink" and all food was "poison dirt" and had determined that starvation was the best way out.

"How are you feeling?"

"Oh . . . better."

"You're eating?"

"Some. I had a very nice dinner last night."

"How's your sleep?"

"Much better, Doctor."

"Good." While talking I slipped the tourniquet around her arm, rubbed soft old flesh with an alcohol pad, and wriggled a butterfly needle into the vein at the bend of the elbow, securing it with tape. Just like being an intern again. Mrs. Goldman made a slight whimper but otherwise lay still. Across from me ECT Mary was checking her pulse and blood pressure, and at her head Dr. Rickey, having finished his squirting, now held in his hands a black face mask, which he flexed to soften, then attached to the ventilator. He puffed it a few times.

"Ready," I said.

"Okay." He leaned forward over Mrs. Goldman, attaching the first syringe to the butterfly, and pushed the medicine. In a few seconds the old lady's eyelids slipped down across her pupils. He took another syringe — the first contained a barbiturate, this one succinylcholine, a neuromuscular junction-blocking agent, and slowly pushed its contents in; within a few seconds she had stopped breathing. He took the black face mask, put a few fingers under her chin, and lifted her head back to open the airway, then puffed up her chest with air.

The succ circulated through her. You could see it, starting at the face and moving down, fluttering her muscles in bursts, leaving them flaccid.

"It's in her calves," I said. Fluttering contractions and releases, a dysphonic, silent wave as blood slowly progressed down her old legs. Finally you could see it arrive at the bottoms of her feet, shaking rivulets that flowed up to her toes, which trembled for a moment, then went. "She's ready."

ECT Mary moved around Rickey, in her hands a big clamp with the electrodes attached; it led to the machine, the old one, a black box that looked as though it belonged to a TV repairman. It rested on top of the sleek new machine, which had buffed aluminum dials and the capability for recording EEG and EKG and for delivering unilateral stimulus and which, unfortunately, had been broken for months — the repairman hadn't shown up. Mary smeared white conducting cream onto the calipers and set them against the old lady's boxy temples.

When I pushed the button nothing happened.

"Should I go again?"

"Wait," Mary said.

Down at her feet you could see slight tremors, then her toes began pointing down, forced by polar current away from her body.

"She's in."

"It's a good one."

We waited. Rickey breathed her, Mary took vital signs; I did nothing until she came out of it and started breathing on her own; then I took her chart and sat down to write my note.

ECT #5
   Pre VS: BP 160/80 P 90   Meds: Atropine 0.4 mg IM
   Post VS: BP   P   Secobarbital   mg IV
           BP   P   Succinylcholine   mg IV
   Tx 160 v. × 0.75 sec
   Bilateral response. Patient had a well-modified tonic clonic
   seizure without complications.

"How much did she get?"

"One forty and sixty," Rickey said.

I wrote numbers in the blank spaces and signed my name.
Mrs. Goldman rolled over on her side. Mary put the siderails
up.

I opened my cup of coffee and drank. In a few minutes,
when Mrs. Goldman was breathing properly, we'd draw the
curtain around her and the next patient would come in. Then
the same routine, the IV, the medications, the black face mask,
the watching for fasciculations. Pushing the button. The seizure. Sometimes so well modified as to be invisible, sometimes not. I hated it. It was an easy way to spend the morning,
true, but the idea of shocking the brain — even though it so
clearly worked I didn't like it. Barbaric, archaic — was that
it? I couldn't really say why I hated being there so much. I
knew every justification for ECT: that it worked fast, that for
someone with a malignant, intense depression it was humane
and effective, that it had fewer side effects than the medications and so was good for the old and the sick. I knew all the
reasons. The history, the neurobiology. Everything. But still I
hated it, this month of what Rickey called "bake and shake."
Rickey seemed to like it, though — putting people under,
breathing them.

I wondered how I'd get the prince to agree. We'd gone over
him in morning rounds, Dr. Brauett, our unit chief, talking
about major affective disorder, depressed, with psychotic fea-

tures; we'd debated phenomenology, mood congruency or incongruency of symptoms, whether it was more likely unipolar or bipolar illness. But I found myself thinking about the prince in a different way, as a character of Mann or Lampedusa, a nobleman in exile, subject to fits of melancholy, this time progressing to madness. His own wealth reproached him, as did his title and the elegance of his life: how could he be so miserable, he asked Kohlman, in a world that was so much more infinitely miserable? He had been in hospitals in Switzerland and France and Austria for sleep cures and hydrotherapy; now he worked in a small foreign bank, which had made some bad loans, the baroness said. The prince, who was held responsible, was demoted but could not quit, and he became terribly depressed, shrinking from food and sleep. Two days ago he had put a loaded gun to his head.

"Doctor?" ECT Mary stood before me. "You done with Mrs. Goldman's chart?"

"Sure. I . . . I just need her last vital signs."

"BP one fifty over eighty, P eighty."

"Okay." I handed the chart to Mary; she tucked it under the corner of Mrs. Goldman's mattress and pulled the curtain. Mr. Donovan came in.

"Mr. Donovan," said Mary, "just bring your legs up . . . That's good . . . Now turn."

I approached him. "Hello, Mr. Donovan. How're you doing today?"

"Terrible," Mr. Donovan said.

"Can Mrs. Goldman go up now?" the aide asked.

"Give her another few minutes."

I picked up the rubber tourniquet, the alcohol pad, the butterfly in its soft plastic box from which I pulled the paper seal. I wrapped the tourniquet, waited for a vein to rise. It was easy to give in to despair here, working with such unhappy, miserable people, or to become ironic and mocking, because the human creature seemed so poorly designed, inclined to fits of self-destruction — cruel, selfish, miserably pleasureless, absurd. You could shock and push pills and do therapy as much as you wanted, and what difference would it make? But *that* was absurd, too, because when you looked at them individually there was usually something you could do. A month in the hospital, half a dozen ECTs for the ones who needed it, could make a difference; you'd see the urge for death disappear.

I taped the needle in.

Rickey was reading a Len Deighton book; he closed it and stuffed it into his back pocket.

"Okay, old man, you'll be asleep in a minute," he said.

And we began again.

The baroness was waiting when I got back to the floor. She was one of those women you see in Manhattan and nowhere else, materializing from taxis, walking quickly down the street with small dogs and large, shiny packages. She had fine, dyed blond hair and wore a shiny red leather blouse and black trousers, and her skin looked hardened and buffed, especially around her eyes and up her cheekbones, as though she was not flesh but had been cast of some light metal alloy.

"I'm awfully glad to see you," she said. "You are the prince's doctor, is that right? I have to tell you right off that we're not the sort of people who go for psychiatry . . ."

There were two other people with her, a tall, sullenly handsome man and a black-haired girl, very beautiful, in white. I led them to my office, where they arranged themselves on chairs, waiting for me to speak.

"Well?" I said.

"We don't think he's getting better here," said the baroness.

The other two were looking around my office.

"We find it so terribly gloomy," said the girl.

"If I were here I'd get even *more* depressed," said the baroness. "Is there another hospital he can go to? Really, he just needs some quiet, somewhere to rest. Maybe he doesn't need to be in the hospital at all ... just a peaceful and quiet place —"

"Where he can pull his head off," I said.

"I beg your pardon?"

"He keeps trying to pull his head off."

"Oh, well, he doesn't mean it," said the man.

"He just needs analysis," said the girl. "Someone to listen to him, and tell him, 'Giorgi, you're really not such a bad man.' "

"Yes, *could* you do that?" said the baroness.

"I suppose you tried it yourself," I said, pushing it back on her.

"Oh, I *did*," said the baroness. "Night and day for the past three weeks. I hardly slept. And all that time we had to have somebody staying with him — you know what he was going to do?"

"So it didn't work?"

"No, it didn't," said the man, before the baroness, almost tearful, could tell me what he was going to do. "Obviously it didn't work at all, otherwise we wouldn't have brought him in here."

"You did the right thing," I assured him.

"You know what he was about to do?" The baroness was crying. The beautiful girl held her hand.

"He knows that already, dear," said the man. "He read the other doctor's note. We're all very upset about Giorgi being in that ... what is it, a straitjacket? And of course we want to help him. We don't like the idea of the E-T-C —"

"ECT."

"Yes, the other doctor was telling me about it. Sounds terrible, really. Isn't there another possibility, a pill or something?"

I launched into my spiel. Kohlman must have had other things on his mind, or been tired, because in ten minutes they had abandoned their ideas about analysis, and I led them over to the prince's room, where he lay, newly released from the camisole. Eddie was right by him.

"I'll be right back," I said, and left them there.

When I returned the prince had his hands on his neck again, and the three of them were trying to coax them away.

"Do you have the certificate?" the baroness said. "Giorgi, the doctor wants you to sign."

"Will it kill me?" the prince said. "Will it blow my head open? Will it make me less despicable and vicious? Already I'm worthless. Why can't you let me alone to take my head off?"

"Let go of your face, Giorgi."

"Giorgi!"

He took pen and clipboard in his hands, staring at them as if they were reptiles.

"Read the certificate, Giorgi."

"We do think it will help you."

"Or blow my brains out?"

"No."

"Do I have to do this?"

"No, of course not. You can refuse. But we think —"

"Giorgi, don't turn your head that way. You may disconnect something . . . What if you become paralyzed?"

"Sign it, Giorgi, *please.*"

The pen hesitated, the pen and paper rose up toward his neck. Other hands brought them down. I still had to call the

ECT committee to approve emergency treatment, call anesthesia, check the EKG and chest film, get all the numbers from
the lab, write a pre-ECT note, call the nursing supervisor. The
pen was still quivering over the paper.

"Giorgi, *please*. He's answered all your questions, *please*
sign."

"I have to leave," I said.

"No! Please . . ." said the baroness.

I walked toward the door.

"Giorgi!"

The pen sank toward the paper.

"Now write," said the baroness. "Just sign your name,
Giorgi, *please*."

"This better go fast," Rickey announced. "I've got a spinal to
do in OB — they just called . . . She's dilated, crowning."

"It won't take long," I told him. It was dark outside the
ECT suite, and you could see the cabs lined up before the
main hospital; the room itself was bright, sterile, polished,
glowing with light.

Rickey flipped through the prince's chart.

"Sixty-one . . . hypertension . . . no other medical problems? Got the consent? Okay . . . Chest film's normal . . .
labs . . ." He looked up. "Okay. So what's this prince stuff?"

"That's what he is."

"No shit. We'll crown *him*," Rickey said.

And the gurney rolled in. The prince was crouched forward
on it, his hospital robe fallen aside, a Poseidon on wheels.

"Where is the electricity?" he said. "I want it on my neck
. . . or my face. Can you give me extra?"

"Just lie back. Lie back, relax. You don't want to tip over."

"Don't you want to see what's inside my neck?"

"Lie back, please."

"Why am I still alive?"

"You'll have to give me your arm," Mary said.

"I have to put a little IV in. Give me the other one . . ."

He lay back, breathing heavily, a muscular, barrel-chested man with a hairy body. There was nothing princelike about him except perhaps a certain angularity of his features, a slant to his graying temples, a prominence of his cheek bones that seemed familial, somehow refined and inbred.

"I am a terrible coward," he said suddenly.

"Now we'll be giving you some medicine that will help you sleep . . . You'll feel very tired in a moment . . ."

Rickey twisted a syringe onto the butterfly and pushed; he took another one and pushed right behind it. The prince's eyes went vacant; his dark lids fell halfway shut.

"Now the succ . . ."

When the moment came the calipers slid off his angled temples; ECT Mary tried to wedge them down but they kept sliding off, into the air. Rickey had to push her away to breathe the prince, who lay flaccid, soft as the just-dead.

"Okay, try again. Hold them at an angle this time."

"I need more paste."

"No — go!"

"We may need more succ . . . Looks like he's coming out . . ."

"Hold the handle up . . . higher. Okay. Stand back. Hands off the table. Go!"

After the button he jerked on the table, biting down with a horrible grimace on the mouthpiece, his arms and legs trembling violently for half a minute, a minute, more, before they suddenly stopped.

"Okay, take it away now . . ."

ECT Mary stepped back.

"Damn," I said.

"Lousy," said Rickey.

"Not very modified, huh?"

"He'll be okay, just a little sore . . ."

"Hope so. What's his pressure?"

"I . . . I don't know. I'll take it now."

"Go ahead."

The next morning there we were again. It was a bright, sunny, and hot late-spring morning, and if you looked out the window you'd start thinking about the beach and running in Central Park and looking at the women. We pulled the windows wide open, and because it was so still and warm put the air conditioner on full blast, too. We did the treatments fast — Mr. Donovan and Mrs. English, whose graham crackers had been taken away, and a new patient, Mrs. Kahan, and then we called the deli to deliver some coffee and bagels, and then we did Mrs. Goldman. We were really hitting it, Rickey and Mary and I, getting them perfectly modified so they barely quivered, just a little curling at the toes. Then the coffee arrived, so we took a break, with Mrs. Goldman in the corner, slowly waking up, drinking our coffee and talking about summer shares in Ocean Beach and Len Deighton and which terrace in the hospital was the best to sit on to get a tan and the biochemistry of depression and why you had to give them a generalized seizure in order for it to work and the earaches of Mary's two-year-old kid.

"What a day, huh?" said Rickey. He sat down on the couch next to me, unwrapped a bagel from its white paper, and tore it in half. "I'll be out of here by three. That's what's nice about anesthesia. Good hours. Plus the money's excellent."

"Sounds good," I said.

"Yeah," he said. "This one anesthesiology resident, graduated two years ago — she just bought a big loft down in SoHo. You make a lot. You work one morning, you get a thousand or two thousand dollars. It's good. It's only inter-

esting maybe five percent of the time, that's the one draw-
back. How 'bout you guys in Psych, how do you do?"

I looked at Rickey for a moment. He chewed on the bagel,
washed it down with coffee. His arms were tanned almost
black. He must sit on that terrace a long time to get that dark,
reading thrillers and looking out at the river.

"It's pretty interesting," I said. "You find out things about
people — I like that. Secrets. What they pretend to think, what
they really think. You figure out why they get in trouble. You
help them. But it's hard. You sit there, you really have to
listen. And you feel a lot of pain."

"Well, I couldn't do that." Rickey grinned. "That's what I
like about anesthesia — they talk too much, you just give them
the gas."

We laughed.

"So what about the prince, what's his problem?"

"Agitated depression. But why, I don't know. I haven't talked
to him much. It's definitely biological, at least part of it —"

"Hey, where is the guy, anyhow?" Rickey called across to
ECT Mary, who was taking Mrs. Goldman's blood pressure.
"Hey there, be a good girl, call upstairs."

Mary glared, but went to the phone.

"He doesn't want to come," she said. "He says it wasn't
strong enough. He wants more volts so we'll blow his head
off."

"Come *on*," Rickey said.

"No, that's what he says."

"He was disappointed by the first one," I said. "He was
expecting a real headache."

"Jesus!" said Rickey. "So tell him we'll give him extra and
get him down here."

"Very funny," Mary said.

"That guy is nuts," said Rickey. "Jesus Christ."

"It is weird to give it to a guy like that," I said.

In a few minutes we heard yelling outside the room, the door was pushed open, and they rolled the prince in. If it wasn't for the yelling you'd almost have thought he was normal, though; he'd shaved and was wearing blue silk pajamas.

"Louder, Prince," said Rickey. "They can't hear you across the street." Rickey always said you could say anything to them before the treatments because they always forgot afterward.

"Hello, Giorgi," I said, and the prince looked at me. "Just lie back and we'll get started in a minute."

"How about plastic explosives," said the prince. "They are very good."

"We don't have any of those here, Prince," Rickey said. "Maybe if you went back to your country you could get some. Don't you have revolutionaries there?"

"Not enough," said the prince. "Can you kill me, please?"

"Glad to," said Rickey.

"Shut up, Rickey," I said.

"Well, excuse me," Rickey said.

I put in the IV, taped it, and pulled the syringe from Rickey's hand. I had had enough of him.

The prince groaned. His eyes dulled.

"Succ," I said. I grabbed the other syringe. "What should we give him, eighty?"

"Give the whole thing."

I pushed it.

"Let's do it right this time," I said. I watched for the ripples in his legs, his feet. "Come on, Mary, get those things ready."

"All *right*," she said.

"Don't you remember?" I said. It was sliding off his slanted forehead again. "Pull your hands up. Come *on*, so it doesn't slide off. Why can't you remember that?"

"So sorry," she said, *"Doctor."*

"Ready?"

"Okay."

I went for the button again.

In the afternoon there was a party for the residents who were leaving. It was up on the unit in the lounge by the river, a bright, airy room, and we stood around eating Entenmann's coffee cake and drinking New York State champagne. The residents, six of us, were grouped at the far end of the lounge, our white coats bright with light from the river. Everyone was talking about how sick they were of the inpatient unit.

"I can't wait to finish up here," Dr. Wagner was saying. "One more week."

"I hate it," said Kohlman. "All these people — their whole lives they've been working on going crazy — and we're supposed to turn them around in a month."

"I can't wait for outpatients," Wagner said.

"Me neither," said Kohlman.

"I kind of like inpatient work," I said. "I mean, I hate it sometimes, but I think I'll miss it."

"What for? Come *on*," Wagner said.

"You're getting too much electricity," Kohlman said. "You're forgetting what it's like up here."

"I know what it's like."

"You like pushing meds, is that it?"

"Yeah, right," I said. "That's it."

Afterward we all walked slowly back onto the unit. After the river lounge it seemed unutterably dingy and dark, and I noticed how stained the carpet was, how battered the woodwork, how stale the air. Right around the corner I saw the prince. He was sitting in a chair, reading. His hair was brushed straight back without a part, and he was wearing a blazer with an insignia on the pocket and neatly pressed tan pants, and holding a slick Italian architecture magazine in his lap. He looked completely out of place here.

"What's going on?" I stopped, dizzy with champagne. The others went on.

"Oh, hello, Doctor," he said. "Do you think maybe I will be going home soon?"

I scrutinized him. It was remarkable, the change in just three or four hours, almost unbelievable. But with ECT sometimes you saw this, it could be this dramatic.

"I'm better, Doctor. You can see. As soon as the medicine wore off I knew I was better. I have a slight headache, yes. But the depression is completely gone."

"You are better," I said. "But it won't last."

"What do you mean?"

"Two treatments aren't enough."

"But I am *completely* better. Why shouldn't I go home today? Or in a few days at the latest."

"Maybe."

"I can sign out, of course."

"You can always sign out," I said.

"You know what it was," he said. "Why I became so depressed? I was trying at the bank to maintain my position, my moral position, after being disgraced. How was I to know the combination of events in Mexico and the recession would happen at a time that the bank was so vulnerable?"

It was bizarre: a madman turned by a few jolts of electricity into an ordinary, troubled man, a man overwhelmed by circumstances, outmaneuvered, exhausted perhaps, but sane. He was not entirely convincing, though; there seemed to be gaps, discontinuities, odd pauses as we talked, which were too quickly interrupted. And he was so eager to convince me that everything was fine that I knew it couldn't be. But he did not sign out, and he agreed to go on with the treatments; he had a third the next day and a fourth two days later. Rickey and Mary and I did him so well his toes hardly curled.

On Friday after ECT I rushed to rounds to sign my patients out for the weekend. We went through passes and medications and weekend problems, and it wasn't long until the prince came up.

"He's had his fourth ECT today," I said. "I don't think he'll be much of a management problem over the weekend. He responded very well to the treatments."

"It *was* unusual," said Dr. Brauett. "Quite an abrupt response after three treatments . . ."

"Two," I said. "My question is whether we should give him more. He's not organic, hasn't had any noticeable memory loss. But since we usually give at least six . . ."

"That's true," said Brauett. "We know there's a certain rate of relapse with too few treatments. And other risks with too many. So what do you want to do?"

I thought a moment. "Stop here."

"Why don't you give one more," said Brauett.

"All right," I said.

"Okay, who's next?" the head nurse said. And we went on to the sadder, more desperate ones.

Monday morning, I was back in the ECT suite, this time with one of the new Twos, Dr. Jerry Cohen, whom I was supposed to train. We were busy as it was, with three new patients and seven old ones, and it was slower with Jerry learning. By the time the prince walked in, with Eddie behind him, it was nearly noon. The prince looked great.

"Hello, Doctor," he said. "You know, I am much better over the weekend. I have thought about what to do with my life — whether to stay at the bank or not." He pulled off his bathrobe and climbed onto the gurney. "And I'm glad this will be my last treatment."

"So am I."

"And I am no more trying to kill myself. It's like a dream I was in, an amazing dream that could not be real, but I see the marks on my neck, so I know it was real."

I introduced him to Jerry and watched as he put the tourniquet around his arm and searched for a vein. He was quick and efficient. I wondered if he knew what he was getting into here. But he was just finishing internship, and maybe this would seem easier to him, here and on the unit. It did, at first, seem easier, but then you saw how sick the people were and how hard it was to help them. Kohlman and Wagner had a point. I would be glad to move off the unit. My new office was downstairs, on a quiet corridor with half a dozen other offices, a white, high-ceilinged room that looked out over the river. You couldn't actually see the river, only the glint of water below, but you could see all the ships going by and the buildings on the other side.

"Now tape it in," I instructed Jerry. "Good."

He reached to Rickey for the syringe.

"Ready to start?" Rickey said.

"Let's go," he said.

"He's a strange guy, the prince, don't you think?" one of the nurses said to me the next morning. "He says such odd things."

"What?" I said. "What is it? Is he depressed again?"

"No . . . I don't think so. Just strange. He and the new borderline were dancing at two in the morning, and he was saying he was going to make a film about his experiences."

"Dancing?" I said.

"Yes, dancing," she said. "He's kind of hyper."

"I knew it," I said. "I knew we shouldn't have given five."

He was in his room, packing a large leather bag with clothes. Things lay all over his bed and the floor, and balanced on one of the posts of his bed was a chessman, a black knight.

"Hello," he said. "Oh, how glad I am to leave. It was really a marvelous experience here, but now I have to get back to work. We're going to reorganize the bank totally, and I need access to the computer system." There was a sort of glaze over his face, and to his motions an activity that at first glance seemed cheerful, but on closer view was something else.

"I see," I said. "Sounds like you have a lot to do."

"An enormous number of things. Now I've wasted an entire week here and things may have slipped from my grasp. You understand how impossible it would be to reorganize the bank from inside the hospital."

He went on about the bank. I listened, waiting for a pause.

"You know, of course, today is *my* last day here," I said.

"Oh, I know," he said.

"Do you think that might have something to do with . . ."

He looked at me as if I were insane. "No. Of course not. It is just that I am better. Perfect. That's all."

At eight that night, after rushing all day to write my off-service notes and introduce my patients to Dr. Cohen, I finally had a moment free to review the chart on a new admission, who had arrived four hours before. But Dr. Brauett was at the nurses' station, wanting to talk.

"What about the prince?" he said.

"Hypomanic," I said. "One of those patients where ECT precipitates a reaction, probably an underlying bipolar picture —"

"Ah. And what do you intend to do?"

"He wanted to leave, but I convinced him to stay, and —"

"Chemotherapeutically."

"I've started Lithium. And we've got prn's of Haldol in case . . ."

"Good."

I got up to go toward my new admission.

"Oh, by the way, here's your evaluation for the year," he said. "A copy of this goes in your folder."

I opened the envelope and glanced at what he thought of me.

"Do you want to discuss it?"

"I . . . not now. I've got too many things to do."

"I have a few minutes."

I put it back in the envelope. It said things I knew too well were true, but would rather not think about now.

"Maybe some time later." I went to see my last admission of the year.

"I just wanted to talk to you about the prince," Jerry said.

"He's still there?" It was three weeks later, and I had been in my office, waiting for a patient to arrive, when Jerry telephoned me.

"Not exactly. He *was* here, but he wandered off the unit. We can't find him. He wasn't ready to leave. We're trying to decide what to do."

"I thought you were going to discharge him the first week."

"We were, but he was too shaky. He had trouble with the Lithium, a DI-like syndrome, and we had to work that up . . ." He went on, talking about Lithium toxicity and organicity. I could hear in the background the sounds of the nurses' station, someone repeating the word *medication, medication.* In front of me, out the window, I looked at the greenhouse that was going up, blocking my view of the river. Its walls weren't clear, they were translucent, corrugated plastic that was bent over a metal frame. It was strange how from down here it was as though the unit and all its craziness didn't exist, as though the miserable, the suicidal, the murderous, all who oscillated helplessly through states of misery and elation, did not and never had existed.

"Poor guy," I said. "I knew he'd have trouble with it."

"Who would know him?" Jerry was saying.

"I'm sorry?"

"Well, he's *gone*. We have no idea where he wandered off to —"

"Have you tried the baroness?"

"We can't locate her," he said. There was a pause. "Do you think he's really a prince?"

"Oh, he's real."

"You think so?"

"Absolutely."

"It's not just some grandiose delusion? And what about the bank? You think he works at the bank, too?"

"What do you mean? I thought this was pretty straightforward. You should be able to check that out."

"We called the bank — they don't know anything about him. We think maybe he has something to do with drugs. Did you ever send a drug screen on him? How well did you know him, anyway?"

Inside the greenhouse a hazy figure walked by from right to left, stopped, raised a hand. Then there was a banging sound, half a dozen times. Then the figure moved to the right, past my window, disappeared.

"I knew him . . . When he came in he was very crazy. Very depressed. But I never . . . never had any reason to doubt his story."

"Well, now he's gone. And we're trying to decide what to do. We don't think he's suicidal, but he's just so unstable . . . It's weird; everything he told you was wrong. Or *maybe* wrong. We just can't tell."

"Well, I don't know, either. Let me know what happens, okay?"

"I wish we knew something about this guy."

Jerry hung up. I wished I did, too, but I guess I didn't. You could think you knew somebody from what they said, but then one thing could happen and you'd find yourself with nothing but fragments, lies. It didn't make sense. The prince *had* to be real. I wondered where the hell he'd gone.

Witnesses

IT IS a semiprivate room set up for burn care. Curved heat shields draped with cotton blankets hang over the beds, monitors blink from the walls, fluids drip from clustered IV bottles through tangles of plastic tubing. The two men here are naked, scraped raw. Their pain stops me, fogs my glasses, raises up sweat between my shoulder blades, under my mask and gown, its presence as strong as the dead-flesh smell that permeates the Burn Unit and spreads through the outer hallways, past the Surgery Library and the Conference Room, so you begin to sense it even from the elevators.

Two men. One is black, heavyset, with a shaved head. He could be eighteen or fifty. His legs are charred, and you can see the small bones of his feet. He is crying in pain. The other man is lean and once was white. A sardonic grin is baked onto his face. His fingernails are charcoal black, and his scorched trunk glows iridescently with Silvadene cream. His arms, they say, are deep. They are swollen like sausages. He is Billano, the Witness. His lashless eyes watch me advance.

I remind myself that there is work to do. I'm the only Psychiatry resident in memory who chose to work the Burn Unit. Now I question my judgment.

I introduce myself.

"What do you want?" Billano says. He is trembling violently.

Jarvis called me here. Jarvis, one of the Surgery residents, paged me at 7:00 A.M., saying something I couldn't follow about closed-space flash burns, transfusions, nadir sepsis, competency, something about a witness.

"Witness?" I asked Jarvis.

"I think maybe he's a Witness," he said. "Jehovah's Witness. Because he's refusing blood products on principle. And we've got to raise his crit before we can debride him. Dr. Whiting wants you to come declare him incompetent so we can go ahead with surgery."

"Is he —" I said.

"Got to go. Just put it in your note, okay?" He hung up.

I phoned my Burn Unit supervisor, Dr. McFarrell. We don't determine competency, McFarrell said. We just determine if the patient understands. Does he know why transfusions should be done? Why's he refusing? Is he psychotic? Delirious? Write it all in the chart, documenting mental status. Don't let the surgeons pressure you.

Billano says something.

"What?"

"I'm cold."

"He's cold," I say to the nurse.

"I'll fix the heat shield in a minute," the nurse says.

He's trembling something awful. I say who I am again. I ask how he got burned. He starts telling me.

He is a firefighter. A tenement building was ablaze. Arson. They chopped their way in with axes. He was dragging a hose upstairs; he could feel the heat under his boots. He had a feeling he shouldn't be rushing up there so fast. He tested the treads and kept going. On the landing, something gave. Then he was hanging head-down in flames. Everything was fire. His buddy, behind him, was trying to lift him out. That is all he remembers.

He shakes harder, talking, the horror returning. The room seems to fill with flames, an inferno worse than a Puritan's most gruesome vision of damnation. What was it: a sinner in the hand of an angry God? My face is seared by his talk. No, Billano tells me, he's no Jehovah's Witness, but he doesn't want blood. Or surgery. He knows the odds. He's set in his mind. I try to work some doubt into him, and for a moment he seems to be hesitating, reconsidering. Then he stops me.

"Too much pain," he says. "I can't talk anymore."

"Is it bad?"

"The worst . . . worst pain in the world. I wouldn't wish it on my worst enemy. It doesn't stop. It's horrible."

"Does the morphine help?"

"Not very long. They won't give me enough."

"I'll check that out," I say, and flee across the room to the desk, where I can hide behind medication records, flow sheets, the chart. I write a quick note — he seems to understand his decision, he also needs higher doses of narcotics — then pull off mask and gown and paper shoe covers and rubber gloves, stuffing them into hampers. I hurry out to the hall.

"How do you find it so far?" says Dr. McFarrell. McFarrell, a plump, loose-jointed man who walks with a shambling farmer's gait, has an intent, somehow irritating way of observing you.

"I feel like I'm not getting anywhere," I say. I could tell him I feel in shock since I've been here, that my whole life's awry, that I dream of flames, that I wake to see if my skin, too, is charred; but instead I just tell him about Billano, whose hematocrit drops every day, who may go into septic shock any moment. I've talked to him, his wife, his fireman buddies; no one seems to be able to change his mind.

"Why's he refusing it?"

"I . . . I'm not sure. I haven't been able to get that out of him."

"Is he afraid of something?"

I think a while. "You know what it is?" I say. "The pain. I just get so freaked out by their pain I can't think straight. They're clearly not getting enough analgesia. I keep putting in my consult notes to increase morphine, increase Levo-Dromoran. They do for a day or so, then it's down again. I tell them what the literature says: the patients won't get addicted, they generally won't have respiratory depression. I even put reprints in the charts, but nothing's changed."

"Why do you think that is?"

"I don't know. Habit maybe. But it seems completely irrational to me."

"It does seem irrational," says Dr. McFarrell. "We can talk about it some time if you're interested. The thing is, burn patients don't *have* to feel any pain. And you're right, they won't get addicted or overly sedated, even with very high doses of morphine."

"So what's the reason?" I ask.

McFarrell observes me. "Watch for it on the unit. See what you come up with," he tells me. He hoists his plump legs up on his desk and looks at me between his feet. "Go back to Billano," he says. "Try to find out why he's refusing."

"I'll give it a try."

"Anything else on the unit?" McFarrell says.

"In the same room, there's a guy with burned legs. A schizophrenic drug abuser. Walked into a trash fire, thinking he was Mr. T. — you know, from the TV show."

"What are you doing for him?"

"Got a history from his father and his social worker, re-started his Thorazine. He's got an even worse pain problem than Billano — screams all the time. He's driving everyone crazy."

Others on the unit include an alcoholic who fell asleep on a couch, with a lit cigarette in his hand, and a vagrant who was robbed, then set afire under the Brooklyn Bridge, and an auto mechanic burned on his arms and chest when a carburetor exploded.

"You know what's incredible?" I say. "Their stories. The way they compulsively retell the story of how they were burned, the way they remember every detail, and the way once they start talking you can't stop them. It's like some basic physiological process, a biological need to bear witness."

"I suppose it must be boring," McFarrell says, "to sit there and have them go through the events."

"Just the opposite," I say. "It's terrifying, but it's fascinating."

McFarrell shrugs. Maybe I'll find something on the Burn Unit that interests me, he says, as though he doubts my word.

"Why are you back?" says Billano. "I don't want to talk to you. Go away."

"It's important," I say. "I need to understand something."

"What?"

"Why you won't let them do the transfusions."

"I already told you."

"No you didn't," I say. "You're not telling me something. I can tell you're holding something back."

There's a long, long pause. "It's because I don't want to get grafts again," he says finally.

"Again?" I say.

"Yeah. I burned myself a couple years ago with gasoline

and they grafted my leg. It was . . ." His crusted eyes glisten. "I'd rather die than have it again."

"How can that be worse than . . . than all this infection?"

His horrible death mask of a face moves with something like emotion. His breathing is ratchety from inhalation burns — it's amazing he made it off the respirator — and it gets faster and faster, until he's heaving like a rusty old bellows. "I've been here for weeks," he says, sobbing. "Nobody, *nobody*'s talked to me, except to tell me I need the transfusions. I can't stand it . . . I keep waking up at night, I see myself hanging in the flames, I keep trying to pull myself out of there, then I stop, I just let myself burn. What kind of life am I going to have if I look like this? I can't even move my hands. I want to die."

"How do you know how you'll look?" I say. But seeing him, I wonder, too. What kind of life? How will he ever walk the street? Maybe death is better. But I'm bound to state the contrary; I'm the doctor. "You've got to let them try the debridement."

"I can't take the pain. They're going to take skin from my legs, and that hurts even worse than the burns. I'm not going to let them do it."

"What if we get you on more pain meds?" I say.

"You promised that already."

"But if I can really get them to *do* it."

"I don't know."

From the next bed there's screaming. Mr. T., as they call him, has pulled his arms free from the restraints and is pulling desperately at the yellow mesh on his abdominal graft sites. The nurse motions me over.

"Be right back, Mr. Billano," I say. "Think about what I said."

I go around to Mr. Thompson's bed. Thompson's burn

pattern is almost the opposite of Billano's: whereas Billano is burned from his head down to his waist, Thompson is burned on his feet and legs. Stoned or drunk, Thompson was convinced he was invulnerable, and to prove it, he walked into a fire. Anyhow, that's the story he told Susan, the resident who had been assigned to this service before me. When I first came by he was delirious. Now there's a different problem. He's getting sixty milligrams of morphine every two hours, a huge dose, which helps him for an hour or so, but then he's screaming again, and, worse, peeling away the grafts. I hold his arm away from the yellow mesh while the nurse ties his restraints back to the side of the bed. Not exactly in my job description, but on the other hand, I never knew that psychiatrists might end up pushing morphine either.

"My feet are burning!" Mr. T. says. "Do something!"

"I don't know what the hell we can do for you," I say.

"It *hurts!*" he screams. His brown, frightened eyes tremble before me.

I feel overwhelmed.

"We'll wait a while and recrop his skin and autograft him," Dr. Whiting says. "How's he taking calories?"

"Twelve cans of Sustacal in eight hours," says Jarvis. "A Burn Unit record."

Everyone laughs.

We're all at Friday noon conference, in a room opposite the Surgery Library: residents in greens, with shoe covers still on and masks hanging from around their necks, the two Burn fellows with piles of reprints, the two social workers, the nurse-epidemiologist, Dr. Whiting, one of the unit chiefs, the plastic surgeon, half a dozen nurses, the occupational therapists and the physiotherapists, and me, the Psychiatry consultant. We're surrounded by food from the deli — sandwiches, cartons of yogurt and cottage cheese, chicken legs in tinfoil, plastic tubs of pasta salad. Jones, one of the residents, is drinking a can of Sustacal.

"Next patient," says Whiting.

Jarvis presents. "Okay. Mr. Billano. Thirty-four-year-old with fifty-four percent deep second- and third-degree burns from closed space flash fire . . . Had neutropenia so we stopped the Silvadene. He's been intermittently hypothermic. Needed excision of his arms, but his crit was falling and he'd been refusing transfusions —"

"Just a second," says Whiting. "Let's hear from Psychiatry."

"I was called in to see him regarding competence," I say. "He did seem to understand the issues. He was refusing transfusions all last week, but he finally changed his mind and agreed to surgery."

"Yeah," says Jarvis. "We got the consent Friday, gave him three units of packed cells and debrided his arms."

"How's he look post-op?"

"Stable: pO_2's ranging from 57 to 76, with pCO_2's in the 45 to 55 range. Been afebrile for two days."

"He still on triple antibiotics?" Whiting asks. "Jones, wake up."

Jones, one hand on his can of Sustacal and the other on his forehead, was dozing off.

"What's that?"

"Billano. His coverage."

"Triple antibiotics. ID wants to continue it for eight to ten days. Their concern is Serratia might blossom in his lungs."

"Okay, let's move on."

"Next is Mr. Thompson," says Jarvis. "He's our thirty-one-year-old model citizen who walked into a burning pile of garbage. He has forty-eight percent third and seventeen percent deep second on his lower extremities, right hand and left flank. His hand's pretty good, but most everywhere else he's tight and he's deep."

"Any hope for his legs?"

"Not really. A little budding on the medial aspect of the left thigh, but otherwise just deep, dark eschar. He's looking at bilateral AKA's at best. Also, he's screaming in pain all day and pulling off his flank dressing."

"Psychiatry have anything to say about that?"

"Yeah. He was a narcotics abuser prior to admission. I've suggested that he be started on methadone, thirty mg a day, and —"

"Jarvis?"

"Okay," says Jarvis. "We'll try it."

"All right, let's move on."

After Mr. Thompson we discuss the other model citizens on the unit. There's a junkie who was sleeping in an abandoned building whom some kids set on fire, the alcoholic with the lit cigarette and one who blacked out against a steam pipe, a hooker whose pimp threw acid on her, and a bookie whose place was firebombed after he fell behind on payments to the mob. They're people who might have tumbled out of *Last Exit to Brooklyn* and been ignited by Céline.

"How about Mr. Paqmhi?" He's the couch sleeper, an Iraqi.

"Nursing's been having problems with the decubitus."

"You getting him on the tilt table?"

"Thirty degrees for thirty minutes. He's tolerating it real badly — screams more than Thompson."

"Psych, could you look at him, too?"

"Okay," I say.

"Social Work, any progress with his dispo?"

"I've been calling every day," says the social worker. "I don't think they like burn patients —"

"Keep calling them," Whiting says.

Tom, one of the nurses, pokes his head in to say that the

surgeons are needed back on the unit. Whiting stands, then Jarvis and Jones, and in a second they're all gone.

I walk back to the unit with the social workers. We pass the front rooms, where patients are moved when they're healthier and closer to discharge. A nurse in cap and gown is carrying a two-year-old baby who has yellow mesh across her face, shoulder and half her back. Drano was spilled on her, no one knows quite how. Deep second, some third. Mr. Washington is being pushed in a wheelchair toward the shower room. Muted yelling comes from the room next to the nurses' station, where Mr. Paqmhi and Mr. Hilber are. No one can stand to go in there. The surgeons call it the grenade room. Mr. Paqmhi wails constantly. Hilber, the vagrant who was set on fire, is constantly trying to assault the nurses and physiotherapists.

I sit in the nurses' station, flipping through Mr. Paqmhi's chart. He's my next consult, but I'm in no hurry to get into that room. The clerk is talking on the phone to a reporter.

"No, I can't tell you if that person's a patient on this ward. You'll have to contact Patient Information . . ."

I'm dawdling. I should be in there with Paqmhi. I should check out how Billano's doing post-op. But something else is on my mind. I haven't thought about it for years.

I was six, maybe seven. This was back in Ohio. One night I was supposed to go across the street for a sleepover with my friend Andy White, but he wanted to come over to my house instead. We argued; he won. Around nine o'clock, as we were getting ready for bed, my mother screamed, and we came running. Across the street the Whites' house, a pretty gray house with a slate roof and a bright red door, was filled with flames, flames that crackled through the windows, filling the street with dancing shadows so the tall sycamores out front seemed to be in flames, too. Andy and I, in pajamas, watched as fire trucks arrived, as firemen dragged hoses across the street, drove their hatchets into the front door, and disappeared inside. Mrs. White, hysterical, pounded on our front door. She'd been down the street at a neighbor's, and for all she knew we were trapped in Andy's room. The next morning, smoke was still rising from the roof.

A few weeks later Andy and I went into the blistered hall-ways, which had the sour smell of wet ashes. We walked across a door that spanned a hole burned through the second-floor landing, and we stared into the floorless shaft that once was Andy's room. In the TV room, Andy's comic book collection was charred, the telephone on which we might have tried to call for help was melted, the receiver fused to the dial. It was a year before the Whites moved back, and a lot longer before I stopped having nightmares, a lot longer before, lying in bed in my third-floor room, I stopped imagining that the shadows I saw were smoke, the lights that moved across the ceiling not the glare of headlights but the walk of flames, before I stopped waking, convinced that I was trapped. Many times I'd lie there and think I heard my mother's voice calling to my father, the Whites' house is on fire, and I would almost hear it as the White House being on fire, and imagine President Kennedy and Jackie and Carolyn and John-John running for safety. Eventually it became almost an entertaining exercise to imagine any house, no matter how solid and dignified, bursting into flames. For the rest of our friendship, Andy and I were always playing with fire, dousing model airplanes with glue and setting them ablaze, dropping plastic soldiers into the flames, focusing the sun's rays with magnifying glasses on leaf piles until a puff of smoke became a yellow flame.

I'm not doing my best clinical work on the Burn Unit — I'm not really *there* with patients. And when I leave the unit and go home, I feel flattened, dulled. I don't enjoy things. Even with Billano, whom I see every day, I feel at a distance, unable to give him much comfort. I know I'm helping him: he's survived the operation, they've increased the narcotics so he's in less pain, but beyond that I'm not doing as much doctoring as I could. That's a terrible feeling. Maybe I'm still not sure I got away unburned. Witnesses, survivors, I know, often have as much dulling of the senses, as many nightmares, as many flashbacks, as much inability to get on with life as the injured themselves. That's true in any plane crash, any nightclub fire, any terrorist attack. But I don't know. Maybe that's just my excuse.

I put Paqmhi's chart back in the rack and take gloves and gown and head cover and shoe covers and mask off the cart in the hallway, then push my way into the grenade room.

A few days later Jarvis comes in while I'm talking to Billano. Billano's doing much better. His face is no longer entirely blackened, but is covered with tiny red dots, skin buds, which in some places — around his ears, under his jaw — are actually starting to meld together. Confluence. His arms have long surgical incisions on them, and much of the dead flesh has been cut away. They are stretched away from his sides, held by braces. His hands are spread wide on splints, each finger held tight by a wire glued to a fingernail. He's always working with the physiotherapist, moving one finger at a time. The nurse, across the bed, is changing dressings, and Billano is mumbling something. Flames, he says, he's seeing flames, he's hanging head-down in them, please, please, would we pull him out.

"What do you think?" Jarvis says.

We both step away from the bed, surgeon and psychiatrist, the two of us identically dressed in gown and mask and gloves. Only our eyes are visible.

"I think he looks great," I say. "He's obviously delirious at the moment, but that should resolve as soon as he becomes afebrile. I'm amazed he's alive."

"Me too," Jarvis says.

There's a long pause. We watch Billano. Then we turn to Mr. T., who is propped up in bed, his blackened legs showing. His toes, the nurse told me earlier, have been dropping off on the floor. He's pursing his lips, breathing rapidly, sort of puffing.

"He's breathing funny, isn't he," I say.

"He's always doing that," says Jarvis. "D'you ever see psychogenic hyperventilation?"

"Psychogenic?"

"Well, there's nothing physically wrong with his lungs. He just starts breathing that way whenever you talk to him."

"It doesn't sound psychological to me," I say. "How are his chest film, his blood gases?"

"We checked them a couple days ago; pO$_2$'s a little low — mid fifties — but there's no infiltrate."

"Maybe you should check them again," I say.

"Sure thing," Jarvis says.

Then I'm beeped for an off-the-floor consult. It's a thirty-year-old stewardess downstairs in the Medical ICU. Turns out she had a fight with her boyfriend and took a handful of pills. Standing by her bed, listening to her story, I see her smooth, tanned arms, her brown, pretty face, and even though she's telling me why life's no longer worth living, and how she's fallen into a bottomless hole, all I can think is that she cannot be suffering, not really. Only the flayed, the burned, can truly suffer, I think. The rest of the world should shout with joy.

Friday afternoon when I come in, gowned and gloved, to see Billano before the weekend, a half dozen surgeons are there. They're drawn close around Thompson's bed. The heat shield is pushed up and to the side. I make out Jones, who's bent over, trying to put a line in what must be Thompson's groin, but is just a mess of Silvadene and eschar and blood. The foot of the bed has been raised to Trendelenburg position.

Jarvis, arms crossed, stands at the foot of the bed.

"What's going on?" I say.

"Septic shock," he says.

"Shock?" I say. "I was just talking to Mr. T. this morning."

"They crash fast here," he says.

"Oh," I say. I turn to Billano, who is up in a reclining chair. Billano's face has an odd expression; the red mask is tighter, blanker than usual. What's wrong? I say. He stares beyond me; he won't meet my gaze.

"I'm going to die," he says.

"No you're not."

"Just like *him*. I know it." He points over at Thompson. He coughs. "They knew he was getting worse. They didn't do anything. Same thing's going to happen to me."

"You're doing fine," I say. His numbers are good, his grafts are taking, there's just the question of whether they'll have to amputate some fingers on his right hand. He'll live. He doesn't believe me, though, I can tell. Eventually I get up, ready to go.

"Oh, by the way, how's the pain?" I say.

"Not too bad."

"You're not feeling drowsy?"

"No, I'm awake."

"Okay, I'll see you Monday."

"If I'm still alive," he says.

The surgeons have gone by now. The nurse is adjusting Thompson's IVs. A large blue and gray box, a respirator, is parked in the space between the two beds, and the tubing from it goes into Mr. T.'s mouth, down his throat. I stand over Mr. T.

I ask how he's doing. His brown eyes are watching me. I think, though I'm not sure, that he nods okay. At the door, as per regulations, I strip off the gown and gloves and mask and stuff them into the appropriate hampers. Billano is still staring at Mr. T. when I leave. And when I stop Jarvis in the hallway to tell him about Billano's cough, he looks at me as though I'm crazy. "Okay," he finally says, "we'll X-ray him, too, if you insist."

"Did I tell you about Mr. T.?" I ask McFarrell. I'm back in supervision again, in Dr. McFarrell's comfortable office.

"Mr. Who?"

"Thompson. The schizophrenic with burned legs."

"Right. What about him?" McFarrell says.

"Okay, well, he was doing all right at first. Then he developed a weird pattern of respirations that the surgeons insisted was psychogenic and I said was physiological. Anyhow, they finally got a chest film and blood gases, and it turned out he had bilateral infiltrates. They'd just gotten around to changing his antibiotics when he went into respiratory arrest. So now he's intubated and basically looks like he's dying."

"You think they delayed the workup?"

"Maybe I'm not being objective about it," I say. "I really . . . I don't know."

There is a long silence.

"It can happen," McFarrell says, and I'm not sure whether he means my not being objective or the workup being delayed.

I don't know what else to say, so I start talking about pain again, the pain that Thompson was always screaming about, and Billano and Paqmhi and Hilber.

"So far the only one who's actually gotten his narcotics increased is Billano," I say. "And that's because I check the order every day." The other patients lie trembling, bathed in pain, a kind of salve spread around the unit, an invisible Silvadene, on every raw, damaged area.

"You know what I think it is?" I tell McFarrell. "I think the nurses and surgeons are afraid to give enough narcotics because they want to make sure *they*'re not the ones who are feeling pain. If the patients are suffering more than they are, then they know they're okay. It's weird, but that's what I think it is."

I go to see Billano almost every day. His face, sprouting with red dots, now looks as if he'd fallen asleep under a heat lamp for several hours — nowhere near normal, but not a black mask, either. His arms need a lot more debridement before they can be grafted, and still look terrible. He is treated for the pneumonia that is discovered on chest X ray, but doesn't respond well to antibiotics, and for weeks he slips in and out of delirium. He'll be working diligently with the physiotherapist, and he'll look fine, but if you talk to him, he'll tell you that he's dragging a hose upstairs, that he knows he's going too fast. The first time he sees himself in a mirror he starts crying.

Mr. T. is still alive, barely. He lies motionless in bed, not even fighting the respirator, which pumps ten or twelve times a minute. At first he's alert and seems to look around at people going in and out of the room. Or maybe he's listening to his hallucinations, conversing with them. But gradually he becomes more bloated and doesn't look at anything.

One morning I come into their room and both beds are empty.

A nurse is standing by the window, rolling up some gauze.

"What happened?" I say.

"Oh, he died last night."

"What? Both of them?"

The nurse turns to look at me.

"No, not both of them," he says. "Billano's over in the Tank Room."

"Oh, thank God," I say. "You think I could go see him?"

"You might want to wait until he gets back."

"That's all right, I'll go now."

"Suit yourself."

I go down to the end of the hall, to the room which, on other floors, is used as a solarium, where patients sit with their families and friends, a big room with a semicircle of windows from which you can see the river and the bridges and the traffic on the drive. On other floors it's a very pleasant place to be. On this floor, it's filled with three long, stainless steel tanks, with curtains pulled partway around them. Billano is lying naked in one of the tanks, and one of the nurses is standing close, working with a scalpel and forceps on his raw arms. Billano is crying. He doesn't take any notice when I call his name. After a while I leave: I just wanted to see that he was still here.

The unit is quiet over the next month. Paqmhi is finally on a stable dose of pain medications, and he'll be walking down the hallway when I come onto the unit. Billano begins a new series of skin grafts, and soon he's up and walking in the hallway, his arms held away from his body by braces, so he has to turn sideways to let people pass. He's been transferred out of the ICU, down to one of the four-bedded rooms out front, with the less serious cases. His buddies from the firehouse come to visit him every few days. They are big, muscular, clear-gazing men who try to stay cheerful. Mrs. Billano comes in every day, but Billano's afraid she's going to leave him. "Women used to love to touch me," he says. "I had to beat 'em off with a stick. Now I'm like the Elephant Man. They'll run away after just one look."

Finally, in November, he is ready to be discharged. He and his wife have packed some big suitcases full of dressing materials and gauze and ointments, and several shopping bags of splints and tape, and he's given a stack of prescriptions. When I go to see him in his sunny front room, he is adjusting the Jobst garments on his arms. Over his face he's wearing an odd mask with eyeholes, like a ski mask, which is supposed to rub against the new skin and make the scarring smoother.

"I can't wait to get home, Doc," he says. "I've got a lot of projects to start, as soon as I can hold a hammer." He wants to winterize his basement, put new windows in his son's bedroom.

"You know," he says, "I got just one problem. I don't know how I'm going to feel walking the streets with this mask on. People are going to look at me and back away."

"Matt," says his wife. She is a small, dark, sad-eyed woman, who is still pretty. They must have been a great-looking couple once. "You don't know how you're going to look. Maybe you'll look fine."

They both start crying.

I see them all the time after he leaves, because he still comes in for physical therapy. His wife will stop me in the hallway to tell me his progress. His hands are moving much better. He has only a few open areas on his chest, she tells me. The one thing is, he never goes outside, except to come to the hospital. What can she do? Plus he's still waking at night, slapping himself, writhing, screaming that he's on fire. And she, too, is feeling it: she doesn't know if she has the courage to keep going, either. She, too, sees flames in her dreams.

The unit is quiet that month. It's unusually warm for November, and people don't need to use their stoves for heat. There don't seem to be as many arsonists at work as usual, and for a time there are fewer children arriving on the unit burned and terrified. There's not much to report to Mc-Farrell. For a few weeks my visits to the unit mostly involve sitting at the nurses' station, listening to gossip. Everyone's waiting for the weather to break.

Including me. There's too little to do now, not enough stories to hear. Every flame, I've realized, ignites a story; in its telling there's a dispersal of heat, a cooling of the inferno. The compulsion to tell, to bear witness — there's something chemical about it, as though neurons discharge as the story is told. I've become a listener here, a fireman, a quencher of flames. But without fire there's no pain, without pain no stories, without stories no need for an ear.

McFarrell isn't must interested in what I say these days. He's somewhat disappointed in my work on the unit. What's all this about storytelling, is his position. Tell me about diagnoses. Tell me about dynamics. Tell me about neurochemistry. It's no use telling him how flames are the source of literature, how in the telling of stories flames lick up again, engulfing both teller and listener.

Certainly, in many ways, I'm relieved by the empty beds.

Early in December the weather breaks; a clear, cold blue front races in from the north. One day three firefighters are brought in, one with 80 percent burns, two with 50 percent, from a warehouse fire in New Jersey. And a college student whose apartment burned. And two boys whose clothes ignited when they were playing with matches in a closet.

And then, the plane crash. A gushing wind on the Atlantic coast, an engine that failed, a sinking to the runway, a smash and a blossom of flames.

The first warning is at lunchtime, on my way up to the unit, when I pass TV trucks with cameras set up outside the Emergency Room, and Dr. Whiting is talking to a reporter. When I get upstairs, the newspapers are calling.

Then the patients arrive. I am there late that evening, and for many hours the next week, listening to their stories.

"We were falling . . . falling . . . I thought we'd certainly die. I said to my wife, why the hell isn't the pilot *doing* something?"

"The engine . . . I could hear a thump when it went, there was smoke coming from the wing, blue flames."

"An explosion when we hit. And flames. I knew I was dying."

There is an elderly woman, and a couple of college kids, and an old man whose wife died in the crash, and two bankers and a lawyer who had been sitting together. They are jittery, agitated; by the time I see the bankers both of them are hallucinating. No one can sleep. They keep waking up, seeing flames, tearing the dressings off their wounds, screaming in the night.

"I climbed over him," says one of the burned college kids. "The cabin was full of flames. I could hardly breathe. I pushed him down. I stepped over him. I was sure he was going to die because he wasn't getting up. And I left him there."

"I have to tell you what happened," says his buddy, an Irish kid. "It's a miracle I ever got out."

"I have to tell you what I saw," says his mother. "I was at the airport, waiting for them, waiting for them to land . . ."

"What I saw," says the old woman with burns on her leg. "I can't get it out of my mind."

"Oh, Doc," says the lawyer, when I finally get to him a week later. He is burned across the chest and arm. Minor burns, first-degree, but he doesn't want to leave the hospital. "Thank God you came." He starts crying. "I've been here for a week and nobody's talked to me yet. I'm in such pain. Do you have any idea of what kind of pain I'm in?"

"A little," I say.

"You couldn't possibly," he says. "Just stay here for a minute, Doc, *please*. I have to tell you exactly what happened to me."

"Okay," I say. "Go ahead."

Beds

AROUND 4:30 P.M. I rush over to the Outpatient Clinic to pick up the bed list for the evening. I've spent most of the day in the Emergency Room, skipping classes, Grand Rounds, lunch and supervision, and still have two patients waiting for me. So when I get to the basement of the Psych building, all I want to do is grab the list and run, but Millie, who does admitting during the day, pulls me aside.

"There's no beds in the City," she tells me. "Bellevue's full, Met swears they're full; I've had calls from all over, people who want to transfer patients. I tell them we don't have any beds."

"What *do* I have?" I say. As a third-year resident on call, I cover the Emergency Room, seeing patients there, deciding whom to admit and whom to send out. Playing God, as Ann, our chief resident, calls it.

"Not much. Two beds, one on Five and one on Three, but the one on Five is being held for a long-term patient, and the one on Three is for research."

"Any discharges tomorrow?"

"One possible from Seven. But they've got a patient on Medicine who's all ready to be transferred back over —"

"So I can't use the cot."

"Exactly."

"So where *can* I admit to?"

"Well, if you absolutely, positively *have* to admit . . ." Millie goes through the possibilities. There aren't many, and if I *do* decide to admit somebody, I have to clear it with the attending first. "Just don't admit more than one."

"Great," I say. I fold the bed list inside the message book, then remember the calls I haven't returned: a Mr. Diaz from Queens and a Dr. Rabindath. So I stop by my basement office and call. I try Rabindath first, and while I'm waiting, I pull plastic wrap off my ham-and-cheese sandwich — a late lunch.

After several rings he answers.

"Hello? Thank you for calling back," the doctor says. He speaks with an accent — Indian or Pakistani. He says he is at a small hospital in Brooklyn. "I have a patient in my Emergency Room," he says. "You might be interested in him —"

"I'm sorry, I don't have any beds," I say.

"Just let me tell you," he says.

"I told you, I don't have a single bed."

There is a pause. Perhaps he is trying to decide whether to accuse me of lying or whether to go ahead and describe the patient to me — perhaps if I find him interesting, I'll suddenly discover an empty bed. I've been on the other side of this often enough, screaming at the administrator at Bellevue or the resident on call at Jacobi, accusing them of lying, of withholding what I *know* is there, that I feel somewhat sorry for him. So I tell him to call Millie in the morning. Maybe we'll have beds then. He says thank you in a mellifluous Indian tone. I hang up and eat a few bites of my sandwich, then dial Mr. Diaz in Queens.

"Hello, Doctor?"

"Mr. Diaz?"

"Yes, this is Mr. Diaz. Tell me, do you have a bed for my son? He just came back from Puerto Rico, he's a schizophrenic, and he's worse. I think he needs to be in the hospital . . ."

He starts telling me about his son, who has been threatening Mrs. Diaz with a knife.

"Where do you live?"

"Queens."

"Where in Queens? What's the nearest hospital?"

"Elmhurst. But Doctor, I don't want him to go back there; it's a terrible place. Can I bring him to your Emergency Room?"

"I'm sorry, I don't have any beds," I say.

"But if I bring him in . . ."

"Do you live between . . ." I describe our catchment area, a small rectangle of the city.

"No, but why should that make a difference?"

I've explained the catchment areas of New York's psychiatric services a hundred times, and even though I hear the desperation in Mr. Diaz's voice, I can't help feeling annoyed. Why do they always put the blame on us? Why do I have to stand in defense of a system I think is ridiculous? Why do I have to spend my days on call turning away desperate people, sending them to state or city hospitals where the care, though not necessarily lousy, is rarely first rate, or back out to the streets?

"But if I bring him to your Emergency Room —"

"Then I'll have him transferred back to Elmhurst. I'm telling you, sir, I have no beds." I sigh. Mr. Diaz is getting to me, too. I give him Millie's number. If his son can last through the night, maybe we'll have beds tomorrow. Tomorrow. What a softie I've become. I don't know how Millie deals with all

these calls. Anyhow, whatever beds there might be tomorrow — weren't they promised away days ago? The whole system stinks. But I've got patients in the ER. I've got to get
back.

I go upstairs from the basement, just to have the opportunity to go out into the March drizzle. I get paged again and
duck into the mailroom to answer. It's the front desk.

"Doctor? There's a psychiatrist on the line. Wants to know
if there are any beds . . . He has a patient in his office . . ."

I curse. I tell the operator to give him a message — no beds.
But I'm barely inside the lobby of the main hospital when she
calls me again. I ignore her. I stop by the vending machines
to grab a cup of coffee, then walk back to the glass-enclosed
nurses' station of the Emergency Room. By that time she's
paging me on both beepers.

"The doctor wants to talk to you *personally*."

Through the glass wall I see the security guard, heavyset,
bored, standing before room 6, the psychiatric room, keeping
an eye on my patient. A woman who went berserk at work
and was brought in by her boss, she's now lying in restraints
on a stretcher.

"Go ahead."

The doctor comes on the line. He is a friend of one of our
professors, he says, and he has a patient in his office right
now, whom he's going to put in a cab and send here for admission.

"Where does the patient live?" I ask. It's getting a bit ridiculous.

The Village, he tells me. He knows the patient isn't catchment, but his friend the professor —"

"Have you talked with him?"

"No, but I'm sure he'll approve —"

"Well, he doesn't have anything to do with admissions.
Anyway, we don't have any beds. So I suggest you send him

to his catchment hospital." I hang up. I have a feeling I'm not through with this patient, that he'll show up in half an hour in a cab, or wander in at 3:00 A.M. with a note from his doctor, or that his family will bring him here and refuse to budge. This situation is impossible, in some strange way similar to trying to find an apartment in Manhattan.

The woman in room 6 is screaming at the top of her lungs. As far as I can tell, she is convinced that there is a plot against her involving both the city of Brooklyn and the IRS. She stops for a moment when I come in, but when I explain that I want her to sign in to the hospital, she starts up again. I go back out and bother the Medicine resident again. She's been here since I came this morning, awaiting transfer to Metropolitan, the city hospital. Hours ago, when there were still beds, I convinced the Metropolitan resident to take her (my hospital doesn't take involuntary patients). Now it's just a matter of getting medical clearance and rounding up the ambulance attendants.

The Medicine resident bristles when I approach him.

"Do you think you could go see my patient? We're all ready for the transfer if you clear her."

"Okay, okay. I'll be there," he says. "I've got an MI and two asthmas first. These are sick people —"

"So's this one," I say.

He pushes out of his chair and grabs the papers out of my hand.

"I'll see her, okay. Any medical problems?"

"Hypertension, nothing else."

Stethoscope in hand, he goes into 6.

I look for my other patient. A scruffy-looking fiftyish man with a bulging suitcase, a muttering street person, like those you see at Broadway and Ninetieth; I'd passed him on my way to 4:30 report. I don't see him now.

I call the security guard.

"Hey, what happened to that guy?"

"Which? The bum? The paranoid one? He was right here. Maybe he's in the bathroom." Security goes and knocks on the bathroom door. "He ain't in the bathroom. Must have left."

"I told you I wanted him to be *watched*," I say.

Security looks hurt.

The registrar speaks up. "He didn't like all the police here. Said he's going to look for another hospital. He's gone."

"Sorry, Doc," says Security. "I was watching the other one, and he must have gone out . . ."

I go back inside the glass booth. Paul, one of the Surgery residents, is there. I know him from the consults I've done on surgical floors. He's on ER now, twenty-four hours on, twenty-four off.

"That your lady screaming in there?" Paul says.

"Not for long," I say. "She's on her way to Met."

"How do you stand it?" he says.

"Oh, you get to like it after a while. I mean, this isn't much fun, but there's good cases every so often. Sometimes it's pretty interesting." I can tell he doesn't believe me (not with the screams in the background), but the odd thing is that it's true. After eight months of ER call, I've almost gotten to enjoy it. First I hated it, absolutely despised the chaos, the screaming, the threats, the lost patients, the surly, nasty staff, and the horrible, overwhelming feeling that all of New York's craziness is ready to walk in your door. But recently something's changed. The patients see something different in me, too — things they've been saying recently, like I'm the first person who really listened to them, that they feel comfortable talking to me. You can turn people around here, if you really listen to them. People who are getting depressed, going psychotic — like a man about to fall apart after losing his job or breaking up with his wife — you can work out a way for them to stay out of the hospital; you make the diagnosis that nobody's been able to figure out before, sometimes for years; you adjust their medication; you figure what's wrong with their therapy; or whatever.

Not that Paul's listening. He's leaning against the counter, looking at one of the nurses, who is talking to a paramedic about her trip to Barbados. The ambulance drivers come in; they're ready to take my lady. Is she medically cleared?

"Yeah, go ahead."

They wheel the stretcher out of room 6, past the security guard, the registration desk, out the sliding doors to the EMS truck that idles outside. The doors slide open, close, and exhaust fumes waft inside. We can't hear her screaming anymore.

Paul's poring over some X rays. The medical people are talking excitedly about atenolol, a new cardiac drug. I sit.

There's a commotion over by the entrance: ambulance attendants suddenly appear, pulling a stretcher, and there's an urgent call on the overhead page. Suddenly everyone at the nurses' station but me rushes out after the stretcher, which is wheeled into the Trauma Room. There's a man on the stretcher, and they're bagging him as they go past.

It's a long while before Paul returns. By that time I've finished my coffee and been paged twice by the front desk — a lady in a midtown hotel having an anxiety attack, a man wanting to ask questions about his antidepressant meds.

"Yes," I say. "That's expected. That's right. No, it's the usual dose. Okay. No, I know what you mean. Right. Constipation. Yes. Goodbye."

I hang up. Next to me, Paul is furiously writing a note.

"What was it?" I say.

"Gunshot wound. Dead by the time they got him out of the truck."

"What happened?"

"Guy was standing at the entrance to the park, minding his own business, and somebody shot him. Probably one of your patients."

"Very funny," I say.

Things get busy. There's a consult in the main hospital, a suicidal patient on the Ortho floor. The Two on call has questions about a patient who is being rapidly neurolepticized. A new patient comes into the ER. An old man with his wife. He came home from the senior center today and found her standing in front of an open window, ready to jump. She meant it, too. If she had a gun right now, she says. Or if she had pills. Or a knife. Her intent is lethal. It's just too much, she says. Her bowels are rotting. Her brains are putrid. Can't I smell the decay?

She won't sign in. I sit beside her in room 6 for twenty minutes, trying to talk her into it; finally I resort to threats.

"I will. I'll send you to the state hospital if you don't sign in. You're a danger to yourself . . ."

Her husband pleads.

She signs. I finish filling out the papers and call the floor to tell them about her. The nurse answers.

"You can't admit a patient here," she says. "We don't have any beds."

"You have a census of twenty-one. According to the sign-out list you have one bed."

"But that's being saved for a research patient of Dr. —"

"Well, it's the last bed in the house." I lie, but she catches me.

"What about Five?"

"They're only taking long-term patients. Look, I went over it with Millie. You get the first admission."

"Then you'll have to clear it with the unit chief."

The unit chief's not at home. The associate unit chief's not at home. The assistant unit chief is at home, and argues with me for ten minutes before I hang up.

When I bring the old lady to the floor, the nurse won't even talk to me.

"Where's the Two?" I say. "I've got to tell him about this lady."

"Find him yourself," says the nurse.

I tell her where to go.

"You'll be in trouble for this tomorrow," she says.

Half an hour later I admit an alcoholic patient to Five, filling the last bed.

Midnight. I'm home. It's dark, and I'm hungry and exhausted. The newspaper is all over the floor. I find dinner on the stove: chicken in congealed juices, rice, salad wilting in its dressing.

I pile food on a plate and sit on the couch, eating.

Right outside our window is the hospital. Across the street, cancer patients in their beds, pots of chrysanthemums, the red blinking lights of monitors, the tangled lines of IVs. One story below is the children's floor, where bald children sit up in bed. Mothers visit, bringing stuffed animals. Fathers stand at the windows, staring down.

It's a strange view to have from one's living room window. Even after two years, we are not used to it. It is subsidized housing, for house staff, cheap and, by New York standards, spacious. The best deal in town, everyone says. Still . . .

I close the venetian blinds. I sit on the couch, plate on my lap, eating.

It is quiet. Eventually I get up and put my plate in the sink.

I call the front desk. "You can reach me at home," I say.

The front desk says goodnight.

I lie in bed. The crosstown bus rumbles down the block and

pauses in front of the building, idling. The windows shudder in their frames. The bus does not move on.

I lie in bed, looking at the ceiling.

No beds. No beds. It is not always like this. Sometimes we have a dozen beds and no one in the Emergency Room, and Millie will call all over the city to see if anyone wants to come to our hospital. We'll take anything, anyone, then. But most of the time only two or three beds out of a hundred are empty. And you are turning people away, trying desperately not to fill them. Because nothing's worse than having no beds.

No beds.

I try to sleep.

I remember being a fourth-year medical student, doing an elective in Psychiatry in a fancy teaching hospital in the suburbs. It was a big, old Victorian asylum, with brick buildings, rolling lawns, maple and oak trees, paths through the woods. One night I was on call with a resident, and a man came to the hospital, trying to get his daughter admitted. It was a very fancy hospital, so fancy it didn't have an Emergency Room. Walk-in patients came into the administration building, a huge mansion with a winding staircase, and were taken to a small room off the formal living room to be interviewed. The resident and I saw the father and his daughter in there. She was having problems, that was clear. She needed to be in the hospital. But the first thing the resident wanted to know was whether she had insurance.

I was shocked. Who cared if she had insurance? Shouldn't we admit her first, worry about money later?

She did, in fact, have insurance. The father pulled out a card from his wallet, but it was the wrong kind of insurance. The resident told the father that he couldn't admit the girl; the father should take her down the road, to the state hospital. He looked upset for a moment, but he grabbed his daughter's hand, and they walked out of the mansion, across the rolling lawn to their car, and drove away. It was a very fancy hospital.

About 3:00 A.M. the phone rings. It's the front desk.

"Hello, Doctor."

I groan.

The doorman, who is sleeping in front of a flickering TV, wakes with a start when I open the door. Outside, the air is cool, and the avenue deserted except for newspapers blowing past the bus stop. I pull my white coat close and hurry across to the hospital.

The surgeon and the medical resident are sitting at their chairs in the glass station, in the same position as three hours ago. They look stunned, exhausted — poor bastards, they're not allowed to go home at night.

The charge nurse comes up to me. She's in her thirties, with close-cropped black hair and a sensible, sensual Irish face.

"You're not going to like this one," she says.

"How come?" I say.

"Dregs of the earth," she says. "I could smell him from across the room. Carrying all sorts of crap in plastic bags — wouldn't let me take them away."

"And?"

"And what?"

"Is he crazy? Does he need to be in the hospital?"

"Oh! You'll see," she says.

"Where is he?"

"Room six. He's talking to the walls."

"What's his name?"

"He wouldn't tell me," she says. "No ID, either."

I sigh. I'm just about ready to turn around and go home; I couldn't have been sleeping more than an hour. My stomach is sour, my eyes are bleary, and I just as easily could do what

some of the other residents joke about — give him seventy-
five cents for the bus down to Bellevue. Or even four bucks
for a cab. I've never done that, of course, but I've sent a lot
of people out without much more.

He stinks.

The room is full of his odor, a piss-sour smell. He's wearing
about six layers of disgustingly dirty rags, and he *is* holding a
conversation with the walls, specifically with a large grease
spot beside the door. He suddenly starts hopping around as
if he's being slapped, then squats down low to the floor and
bangs his head on the dirty linoleum, hard. I say hello; he
doesn't move. There are deep ugly gashes on the back of his
dirty arms, and his feet are swollen with the beginnings of
cellulitis, but as far as I can see, not enough to justify IV antibiotics. Too bad — just a little more, an open wound, some
cellulitis, a bit of osteo, and Medicine'd have to give him a
bed. And they don't have to worry about catchment.

Looking at him, I'm surprised to find that he's young. Awfully young, with a kid's stubble, traces of acne on his cheeks.
Brown eyes, with an eerie, placid blankness. I search for the
person behind those eyes. Is he scared? I wonder. I try to feel
his suffering, to imagine how horrible it must be to wander
the streets of Manhattan, insane, impoverished, with nowhere to go, totally at the mercy of the worst of the city,
unable even to know what reality is, but I feel nothing. I ask
his name.

"Arkipestipissifullen," he says. He spits at the couch.

"What was that?"

Nothing.

"Is something bothering you?"

Nothing.

"What are you spitting at?"

Nothing.

I try everything I can think of, every interviewing technique, every approach, every question. I do about everything short of crouching on the floor with him, which I might have done if the broad-faced security guard wasn't standing outside watching. Maybe another time I could get through to him, maybe at an earlier hour, maybe if I hadn't been screaming at people all day. But no matter what I try, Mr. Arkipestipissifullen is adamant about revealing nothing to me, not even his name, as if he wants to remain what he seems at first glance, and only that — a grubby street person you might see pawing through a garbage can or sleeping next to a heat vent in the dead of winter. But finally he says something that sounds like Macon.

"Macon?" I say. "Macon, Georgia? You from Georgia? You're from Macon, Georgia, right?" Nothing. "You are, right?"

Nothing.

"Your name's Fullen?" I reach for a fragment from his earlier response.

"Once it was Fullen," he says. "Then it was McDermott. Then it was Swanson. Then it was Arkipesti . . ."

"Right," I say.

This'd be the time for a smoke, if I smoked, or a good stiff whiskey, if I drank whiskey. I leave him chanting "Arkipestipissifullen . . . Arkipestipissifullen" at the grease spot on the wall and go to the phone.

I call Georgia. I must be crazy, especially at this hour.

"Any Fullens in Macon?" I ask.

"Not in Macon," the operator says finally. "But I see a Bill-John Fullen in Jeffersonville; that's just outside Macon."

I call. Fifteen rings before a thick, sleepy voice answers.

"Mr. Fullen?"

"Yeah? What you want?"

"I'm calling from New York. I've got a patient here in my Emergency Room who I think might be a relative of yours."

"Yeah?"

"A kid, about eighteen, nineteen. Brown hair . . ."

"Nope. Never heard of him . . . No, wait a minute, that could be my nephew Bobby." He doesn't sound too happy at the thought. "Bobby . . . he's been in one nuthouse after another. Wacko again, is he?"

"Well, he's . . . he's pretty disorganized."

"Yup, that's him. Wacko. But you don't want to talk to me, you want to talk to his mamma. But his mamma don't have a phone. You give me your number and I'll get somebody to drive on over and take her to a phone."

"Okay."

"May be a coupla hours. She's over to Stroud, that's fifty miles from here."

"Okay. But maybe you can tell me . . ."

Uncle Bill-John doesn't know a whole lot, and what he does know doesn't help much. He's just wacko, Bill-John says. Sometimes he comes back to himself, then he goes wacko again. And when he's wacko you got no choice but to lock him up, that's all there is to it. We'll lock him up, won't we? I don't know is all I can say.

Afterward, from the glass booth, I stare out at the dirty plastic chairs of the empty waiting area and try to figure what I'm left with. Bipolar? Schizoaffective? Toxic? Plain old undifferentiated schiz? Whatever he is, what I've basically got here at 4:45 A.M. is a man who needs a Psych bed when there aren't any Psych beds in town. I've got a problem.

I call Bellevue first.

"We won't touch him," the administrator says.

"You *have* to take him. He's . . . he's an undomiciled male who's acutely psychotic. He needs admission."

"I don't have any beds. I've got people lined up in my ER waiting eight hours to be seen."

"I don't care. You have to take him. You're required by law to take *all* undomiciled —"

"Try Met," he says, and the line goes dead.

I call Metropolitan.

"Where did they find him?" the Met resident says.

I tell him.

"That's not our catchment. That's Bellevue's."

"They just refused to take him."

"They *have* to take him."

"That's what I told them."

"Well, I don't have any male beds, and it's *their* patient. They know damn well it's their patient. Anyway, they just send their excess patients to Kings County . . ."

"Those sons of bitches," I say.

I dial Bellevue again; but while I'm waiting for the operator to page the administrator, I think to myself, Screw it all! Screw it! I know what'll happen if I get through. We'll scream at each other for half an hour, then I'll have to call the chief resident or the medical director, and they'll call the chief resident or medical director at Bellevue, and they'll all scream at each other for a while, and it'll be half a day before Mr. Fullen gets out of that stinking room and sent down to Bellevue. And then they probably won't even admit him. They'll just give him a dose of medication and send him back out. Screw it!

I hang up.

I fill out the papers and go back in. Mr. Fullen is squatting on the floor, in the same position as when I left him.

I squat down next to him, my white coat fanning around me on the floor. Security looks in on us, grinning.

Mr. Fullen hops away, but stops when I call his name.

"I want you to sign in, Bobby," I say. I hop forward one hop and extend my clipboard for him to sign.

We've just barely begun morning report with Ann, the chief resident, in her office, and the Two, and me, when my beeper goes off. I use Ann's phone to answer.

"Doctor, this is the Business Office. You admitted a Mr. Robert Fullen last night?"

"That's right."

"There's some information I need."

"Okay," I say.

"You didn't fill out his address on the admission packet."

"He doesn't have one."

"He's undomiciled?"

"Right."

"And you didn't fill out the type of insurance."

"No insurance."

"Medicaid?"

"No, nothing."

"Is he a New York resident?"

"I . . . I don't know. I think he came into town a few weeks ago."

There is a pause. Ann and the Two are talking about the first admission, the old lady.

"Anything else?" I say.

"The patient is not in our catchment area, and he has no insurance. I don't understand why you admitted him to this facility."

"Because it was the right thing to do."

"But you could have transferred him."

"Oh, I could?"

"Yes." Business Office completely misses the tone of my voice. "He may still need to be transferred."

"Look, I'm sure you people in the Business Office can figure out some way to pay for his stay, if you want to."

"I . . . I don't know, Doctor."

"Christ!"

There is a pause. "Can I go?" I say.

"I will have to put on the form, 'admitted against financial advice.' "

"You do that," I say. I slam down the phone.

"What was that all about?" Ann says.

"The third admission," I say.

"He's a real dirtball," says the Two. "The nurses threw him in the shower before they'd even talk to him."

"What's the problem?"

I explain.

"It's a system problem," Ann says.

"You're telling me."

"We're working on it. We have a committee of all the hospitals in the city."

"Well, you better work fast. We all spend our nights banging our heads against the wall."

The door opens: it's Adam, the Three who is on today. I give him the ER beeper, the message book and the bed list, which he looks at, scowling.

"No beds?" Adam says.

"Nothing at all. No discharges today, and there's one cot filled already. And a couple people scheduled to come in," I say. "Oh, and by the way, no beds in the whole city."

"Oh boy," says Adam. "How was last night?"

"The usual. Oh, there may be a patient on his way to the ER, a young guy from the Village, bipolar, manic —"

"Can we get back to rounds?" Ann says.

"Yeah, sorry." Adam leaves, and I tell about Mr. Fullen in the ER.

"That's nothing," says the Two, "compared to what happened once he got to the floor. I had the worst night of my life."

"Let's hear about it," says Ann.

I sit back and sip my coffee, oddly relieved, almost cheerful, ready to hear tales of disaster.

But I'm not out of it yet. The rest of the morning, there is one call after another. You'd think I'd committed some kind of crime. The unit chief of Three calls me out of professor rounds, upset that I filled his last bed with a nonresearch patient. The assistant unit chief of Five interrupts my long-term therapy case, upset that I admitted a "damn demented geriatric alcoholic who needs a medical workup" to his long-term adolescent floor. During noon conference there's a second call from the Business Office about Mr. Fullen's financial status. As I'm on my way to the deli at noon, Millie stops me to say that, by the way, didn't I know I'm *not* supposed to use cots if there's not going to be another discharge in the next twenty-four hours. And anyway, wasn't it pretty clear that Mr. Fullen didn't meet "cot criteria"? Surely by this time of year I ought to know *that!* And the guy at the front desk keeps beeping me, saying the ER wants me. Come on, I tell him, I'm not on today. Let them talk to Adam.

Then, around three o'clock, during Medication Clinic, the ER beeps me directly, five times in a row. So I answer.

"Hello? This is Dr. Hellerstein. Why do you keep paging me?"

"Hold on."

A nurse picks up. "Hello? We've got an outside call for you."

"I'm not on today."

"They want you. Long distance. Let me switch you over."

"Hello, Doctor?" A woman's voice, with a Southern accent, a white-trash crackle in her throat. "I hear you-all found my Bobby."

"Mrs. Fullen?"

"Yes, that's me. Tell me, do you have my Bobby there?"

I sigh. I look over at my patient, a schizophrenic lady who seems to be hearing voices coming from my bookshelf.

"Did you find him? Do you have him there?"

"For the moment," I say. "He was wandering the streets, completely crazy. Somebody found him and brought him to the Emergency Room."

"He just hopped a bus right out of town," she says. "Last month he left, and we had no inkling where he'd gone to. We didn't know if he was dead or alive." She sighs, as if not sure which would be better. "You'll keep him until he's better, won't you? He needs to be kept for a long while. You'll hold on tight to my Bobby, won't you?"

"For the moment," I say. "For the moment. That's all I can promise."

"May the Lord bless you," she says. "Forever and ever and ever."

The Assistant

IT'S FIVE-FIFTEEN Friday afternoon, and the nurses' station on Eight is a madhouse. It's eighty-five degrees. The air conditioner, jammed into the only window, blows hot air — the compressor's dead. The nurses are finishing up report; the brand-new residents, who just finished their internships three weeks ago, are furiously writing notes; the medical consultant is sifting through a pile of pink paper for a certain lab result. Everyone's talking. The phone is ringing, but the clerk, on the other line, ignores it. One of the nurses is trying to hand out paper cups of pills from a blue plastic tray to patients who are lined up before the door. They look in at us, amused at our craziness.

Then Victor arrives. Victor, our chief resident, is as new at his job as I am at mine. We also started three weeks ago, on July 1, that date when medical students become interns, interns become residents, and residents graduate. Behind him trail the resident on call, the nursing supervisor and a few medical students.

"Hey! Let's have some quiet!" Victor yells.

Everyone goes silent for a moment. But then there's shouting from the ward, and the aides go out to see what's happening, and everyone's blabbering again.

Victor and the resident on call and the students all crowd around Donna, the nurse who's giving report. Bernard and Shriver are on maximal observation, Paul is talking suicide but probably won't do anything, André needs more Haldol. I turn back to the chart I'm trying to review, one of Ellie's patients.

For three weeks I've been assistant unit chief on the eighth floor, an inpatient unit at the best madhouse in the city. According to my job description, I supervise residents and Psychology interns and medical students, run meetings, teach and do research. But so far my job has come down to just one thing: trying to keep Ellie in line. Ellie McDonald, one of the new second-year residents, is impossible. She's blond, pale, a graduate of one of the six-year B.S.-M.D. programs and very, very young, even for twenty-five. Her notes are sloppy, her presentations are confused, she always tries to get someone else to do her admissions, and you can never find her when you need her. Worse, she actually seems to take pleasure in giving you a hard time. And then, just as you're about to bash her one, she apologizes: so sorry you couldn't find me, gee, I really should have told the nurses where I was. It won't happen again, I promise. Sure, Ellie.

"Hey! Hellerstein!" It's Victor. "What's with this new patient hearing commands to kill herself?"

"Which one?" I say.

"Tina something."

"Tina Brown." She's Ellie's patient, of course. "I've got the chart right here. There's nothing about voices."

"Donna says the patient's been hearing commands."

"Well, Ellie presented her at team meeting and didn't say anything about it."

"Did you see the patient?"

"Not yet," I say. Realizing I should have. She could be hanging herself, cutting her wrists, right this moment.

"Where's Ellie?" I ask the clerk.

"I don't know. I just tried to page her."

"Well, she was at team meeting," I say. "Is she signed out for the weekend? Hey!" The residents, Lazlo and Ronald and Jan, look up from their charts. "Did she sign out to any of you?" No answer. "Damn it! Did she ask anyone to cover for her?" They shake their heads.

Victor pushes the door open and strides out onto the ward. I follow. He's furious, I can see, but I'll be damned if I'm going to let him blame it on me. I can't keep my eye on Ellie every minute.

We find Tina in her room. She's a cute little fourteen-year-old, crazy as anything. Victor takes his hands out of the pockets of his grimy white coat and grabs her arm: there's something red on her wrist. He pulls up the sleeve of her gown. It's too red to be blood, too flat. Looks like magic marker. Behind her, on the wall beside the bed, she's drawn crazy graffiti, and weird, sneering faces — a devil, a maddened Donald Duck. Victor, ignoring them, interrogates Tina about her voices. How many are there? Where are they coming from? What do they tell her to do? How'd she get those scratches on the back of her hand?

When he's finished, he glares at me, orders an aide to stay with her, and hurries back to the nurses' station.

There, in front of everyone, he details my failings as assistant unit chief.

"I hold you personally responsible," he says. "That girl could have killed herself. If your residents aren't getting an adequate history, then you should talk to every patient as soon as they get to the floor. Understand?"

I look at Victor. "First of all," I say, "I don't think she's really suicidal."

"I don't want to hear it," Victor says. "We're running late. We don't have time to discuss this. Just get Ellie to do her job, that's all." He turns and leads the Two and the students and the supervisor out of the nurses' station.

"Damn it!" I say. "Where is Ellie McDonald? I'm going to kill that jerk."

"She wasn't hallucinating," Ellie says Monday morning. We're sitting in my office, a tiny room with a linoleum floor and a sink in the corner and a slit of a window showing a gleaming slice of river.

"Then what was she hearing?" I say.

"They weren't real voices. They were parroty sounds — that's how she described them — one in her left ear, one in her right ear."

"They weren't saying she should kill herself?"

"No."

"Did you ask her?"

"Yes. Yes I did." Ellie sits forward and puts her hand on my arm.

"But you didn't put it in your note."

"Because it was negative. Why should I put that in?"

"Because it was on the ER note. You've got to cover your ass." I pull away from her. "Anyhow, where were you? You know you're supposed to sign out your new patients."

"I forgot, okay? I went home and I forgot to sign out."

"You forgot?"

She bursts into tears. She was on call the night before, she says, she'd had practically no sleep, and then she had to admit this patient. It wasn't *fair*.

"But Ellie," I say, "you volunteered. You said at rounds Friday that you wanted an admission because your census was low and you have a lot of discharges coming up."

"So I was wrong," she says. "I thought I could handle it."

"That's understandable," I say. "But the patient's safety is our main concern."

"Okay. Okay, you're right. Just don't get so down on me. Give me a chance, okay?"

She picks up her bulging briefcase and rushes out of my office. I can hear her wrestling with the door to the unit. It slams. A few minutes later I follow her into rounds.

In rounds, I sit between Dr. Blanding, the unit chief, and Roberta, our head nurse. Lazlo and Ronald present the two admissions from the weekend, an old lady with agitated depression and a twenty-five-year-old who abuses cocaine. Then we hear weekend report. One patient cut her wrist on Sunday but didn't require stitches. A patient scheduled for shock treatment drank water at 5:00 A.M. Can he still get his treatment? We go quickly through our twenty-five cases, the nurse reading a brief report, the resident writing orders. I'm a bit nervous as I hear all this news. It's hard to keep it all in my head, to remember the plan for each patient, to think of what we've forgotten. But after a while I sit back and relax. The staff is good. Nothing will go wrong. It's still cool at this hour, and it's very pleasant to be sitting here, in this room along the river, from which you can see the water and the barges and the tankers. After all, this is more or less my operation now. I don't have to draw bloods anymore or sit for hours on the phone or run all over looking for an EKG machine. Never mind that Dr. Blanding's officially in charge: after thirty years at this hospital he's more than glad to let the assistant take over.

Roberta closes the report book after the last patient, and people start leaving.

"Hold on," I say. "Who's up for admissions?"

The nurses and social workers and students file out; the residents stay.

"I have five patients," says Jan. "I'm not discharging till next week."

"I have six," says Lazlo.

"I have five, also," says Ronald.

"Ellie?" I look at her.

"Three. But I don't want to admit any patients today."

"Well," I say, "you're clearly up first. If you can get someone to trade . . ."

No one says a word.

"Looks like it's you, Ellie," I say.

"That's not fair," she says. "I admitted Thursday and Friday. I'm going to be up all week."

"Look," I say, "that just happens sometimes. It happens to everyone. There are weeks when you don't have any admissions. That's just the way it is."

"Why don't *you* admit patients?" she says.

"Me?" I say.

"Yes, *you.*"

I laugh. "Ellie, I can't believe you."

"Really. I'm serious."

"I have enough other things to do," I say.

We have staff lunch every Monday at noon with Dr. Blanding and Roberta and the social workers and me. We usually go down to the elegant dining hall at the research institute. Today, though, we're short on time, so we eat in the hospital cafeteria, a windowless basement. On one wall there's a mural showing the hospital in its various incarnations, from its infancy as a small brick building, to its second stage as a high, dark Victorian building, to its current shape, achieved fifty years ago, a towering neo-Gothic structure, whose peaks King

Kong might easily be imagined to scale in search of Fay Wray. The painting, an idealized view, shows the current hospital right along the banks of the river, as though you might just stroll out to the water's edge for a picnic, without being run over by the careening traffic on the drive or mugged by vandals stripping abandoned cars.

"So, how have the residents been doing?" asks Dr. Blanding.

"Pretty well," I reply. "Ron's having some problems setting limits with his borderline patient. He was seeing her over an hour a day. I really had to get down on him to shorten the sessions. But he sees that she's better when he just doesn't give in to her. Lazlo's still being obsessive. And he's not giving enough medications. Jan is doing great. I don't have any complaints about her."

"What about Ellie?"

"Ellie!" I say. "My God! I don't know what to do with Ellie."

"I just got a call from her this morning," Dr. Blanding says. "She says she's being assigned more than her share of admissions. She wanted me to excuse her from admitting patients today."

"Are you kidding? She doesn't do anywhere near her share. The other Twos are about to kill her."

"So are the nurses," says Roberta.

"How's that?"

"Well, she always writes her orders wrong," says Roberta. "We've gone over the right format a dozen times, but she still leaves things out — whether to give them p.o. or i.m., how often. Then, when you page her, she'll scream that you're interrupting her. Or she won't answer at all."

"Not to mention," I say, "she keeps forgetting to sign her patients out."

"Doesn't she do anything right?" says Dr. Blanding. "I like her."

"That's because she flirts with you," says Roberta.

"She does flirt very nicely," says Dr. Blanding. He seems amused.

"Well, it bothers me," says Roberta.

"I don't care who she flirts with," I say, "as long as she does her job."

"Is she having personal problems?" asks Dr. Blanding.

"I don't know."

"Couldn't we fire her?" says Roberta.

"I only remember firing one resident," says Dr. Blanding. "And that was a fellow who got one of the long-term patients pregnant. It was very embarrassing because the patient was delusional, and she kept telling people that I was the father."

We all laugh. My beeper goes off. It's the unit. They can't read one of Ellie's orders, and she's not answering her pages.

I tell them that it should read 5 mg p.o. or 2.5 i.m. q 2 h prn severe agitation. "Okay?"

"Okay."

"And leave Ellie a note about it," I say. "I want to see her."

When I get back to the table they're still talking about Ellie.

"You know, I think we need a plan for her," I say.

"How's that?"

"Well," I say. "Let's assign one of the nurses to go over her orders with her every morning. Dr. Blanding, every time she calls you to complain, just refer her back to me. And let's keep track of when people can't find her, what the circumstances are. I'll meet with her a couple times a week ... I mean, she can't beat us all."

"Want to bet?" says Roberta.

That very afternoon I find Victor having at Ellie in the nurses' station in front of everyone.

"You don't *think* you write an order," Victor's saying. "You damn well *write* it, and check it, and see your goddamn patient before you change doses."

"What's going on?" I ask.

"You should know," Victor says. "You should be on top of this. It's the same patient. She's having a dystonic reaction right this minute, and we're coming around on afternoon rounds and the nurse tells me there's no order for Benadryl."

"But I wrote the order this morning," Ellie says. Her eyes are full of tears.

"Then where is it?"

"I don't know. It should be in the order book."

" 'I don't know' isn't acceptable," Victor says.

"Hey, Victor," I say. I pull him out of the nurses' station and around the corner, into the dining room, which is empty. Victor clenches his jaw; he's obviously counting the seconds. "I think it'd be better if you backed off."

"How? How's that going to fix this mess?"

"Because we're working on it," I say. "And screaming doesn't help her any. Why don't you go on with sign-out. I'll take care of Ellie."

"All right," he says.

We go back to the nurses' station. I take Ellie with me down to Tina's room. Tina, in a sweatshirt and jeans, is sitting on her bed. She's paler and pudgier than when she came to the hospital. Her head is twisted to the side, and her tongue is stuck in the corner of her mouth. On the table beside her bed is a pile of drawings. The faces are less angry than those she drew when she first came in, and the words in the balloons make some sense.

"Can you straighten out, Tina?" I say. She strains but her head moves only a few inches. "Ellie, test her muscle tone." Ellie reaches for Tina's hand. "No. Like this. Take her wrist in your hand. Hold just above the elbow. And bend back and

forth. You've got to check for parkinsonianism. There's cog-
wheeling, right?"

"Right," Ellie says.

"So go tell the nurse we want Benadryl. Twenty-five i.m."

"Okay." Ellie goes.

"You'll feel better in a few minutes," I tell Tina. "We'll stay
here until you're better."

Afterward, I take Ellie to my office, and we go through the
chart page by page.

"Let's look at today's note," I say. "What do you mean,
'muscle tone normal'? She's had three reactions in the past
twenty-four hours. Is she posturing or really having dystonic
reactions? And 'mental status unchanged.' That's just plain
wrong. She's hallucinating more, she's more delusional, she's
thought-blocking. Is she organic? You don't indicate that
you've even *thought* about these things. And your orders . . ."
I flip through the order sheets, to the most recent set. "Look
at this. You rewrote the orders yesterday but you left out the
Cogentin. Was that on purpose?"

"Yes," she says, blushing. She leans forward, her knee against
my knee, and touches the back of my hand. I pull away.

"It was? I don't agree with it. But if it was on purpose then
you have to write d/c Cogentin. And what about the Benadryl? Same with that. I can't blame Victor for getting upset."

"He really picks on me," she says.

"He does," I say. "But these are basic things. It's not so
hard to do them right."

She leans forward again, close to me, and I pull away again.

"So, are you going to increase the Haldol?"

"I'll do it, but I don't want to."

"You're not in much of a position to disagree," I say. I
close the chart and hand it back to her. "Oh, there's one more
thing, which I don't think you're going to like. This . . . this

touching. I don't know if you do it because you're nervous or what, but I think it makes people take you a lot less seriously."

"Oh!" Ellie takes a deep breath. "Okay." Not looking at me, she gathers her things together and leaves.

"You don't think it's getting better?" I say to Victor at the assistant unit chiefs' meeting. Half a dozen of us assistants meet twice a week to go over the problems on our floors. I'm back at my usual topic.

"Maybe a little," Victor says. "But not fast enough. She's really getting on my nerves. A couple more bad evaluations and she just might get bounced."

"You know what I think," I say. "I think she can handle the work. She's just nervous about taking responsibility for patients."

"You're really giving her the benefit of the doubt," Victor says.

"I guess." I talk about our plan for Ellie, and the other assistants toss in some suggestions. Victor doesn't say anything more about Ellie, so maybe he thinks it's okay. He goes on to talk to the assistant from Two, whose residents are threatening to go on strike.

I suppose I am giving Ellie the benefit of the doubt, because for the next month or so she continues doing fairly lousy work. The nurses still scream at her for her orders; the notes she writes, which I go over with her every afternoon, are still vague; her presentations at professor rounds, which I also review with her, are incomplete and badly organized; and she still does strange things, like trying to transfer a patient with chest pain to the Coronary Care Unit before even getting an EKG, or announcing one Wednesday that she's leaving that afternoon for a long weekend in Florida. But my basic feeling is that eventually she'll be okay, that eventually she'll calm down and start doing decent work. I remember how it was being a Two, suddenly switching from the certainties of medicine, the lab tests, the numbers, the X rays, the magic drugs, to the utterly foreign territory of psychiatry, where your frames of reference are constantly shifting, where there are damn few hard facts, where your treatments depend on how you use your "self," where you can feel like you're drowning in madness, and where if you're angry or preoccupied it can ruin your work.

As a Two I was just about as scared and bumbling as Ellie is. The only difference was that I wasn't the worst resident on the floor — I was the second worst. So I didn't have to go around being blamed for everything that went wrong. The resident who was the worst on my floor *was* blamed, and she had such a miserable time that she almost dropped out altogether.

So in a way I guess I'm easy on Ellie.

And things improved — by November she begins to do pretty good work. The nurses don't hate her anymore. On her birthday Roberta even brings Ellie a cake in rounds. Of course, Ellie's not perfect, but if she tries to start ducking an admission, I just remind her she's up to her old tricks again, and after a few minutes of arguing she suddenly smiles embarrassedly and agrees to take the case.

She's doing well enough that I can be away for a few hours or the entire day and be fairly confident the floor won't be in chaos and Ellie McDonald nowhere to be found when I return. Lazlo is out for two weeks for a knee operation, and Ellie, amazingly, does her share in helping to cover for him. When I take a week off at Thanksgiving, I'm almost tempted to ask Ellie to be acting assistant unit chief, but after one of her sarcastic comments to Roberta I realize that's hoping for too much.

One problem remains, though. Ellie doesn't like letting go of her patients. Unless I keep bugging her about it she won't set discharge dates or find the day programs or clinics or whatever follow-up they need. Dr. Blanding and I have a running argument: Is it because she's too attached to her patients or that she just hates doing admission workups? Either way, it's clear that she keeps her patients for days or weeks longer than they need to be in the hospital.

Tina's the worst. Ellie has become very attached to Tina, who's very playful, always bringing Ellie candy or fruit or giving her funny drawings. And Ellie brings Tina things from the gift shop or the deli. They like each other — that's fine. But now all Tina needs is to be medicated enough to be discharged. It sounds simple. A stable dose of neuroleptics, interviews at a home for adolescents, set a discharge date. But Ellie has found it incredibly complicated. For one thing, Ellie thinks Tina is on too much medication. So she's continually writing orders to lower the dose. When the dose gets low enough Tina becomes psychotic again and does something mildly self-destructive, like scratching her hand, and the interviews at the homes have to be postponed. Ellie increases the dose again and Tina has a dystonic reaction or becomes oversedated. Then Ellie switches to a new medication. And the whole cycle begins again.

One day in December, the third or fourth time this has happened, Tina is put in seclusion for attacking another patient. I've had enough. I corner Ellie after rounds.

"Now what have I done?" Ellie says.

"It's what you haven't done," I say. "Don't you think it's time we got her out of here?"

"She's not ready yet. She's still psychotic."

"Only because you cut down her dose again."

"Well, she's been looking so much better, I thought she didn't need as much. I don't want her to get tardive."

"But she obviously needs that much right now," I say. "You think it's better that she keeps relapsing?"

"I don't know. I . . . maybe if we keep trying other medications we'll find one that works."

"You haven't tried any of them long enough," I say. "You'd have to keep her on one dose for at least a month, but you change every week. Anyhow, there's no reason that has to be done here. They can do it at the group home."

Ellie sits very still.

"What?"

"I don't want . . ." she says. She pauses.

"What?"

"I don't like the idea of her going to the group home. I think it's terrible. She's not going to have a family there. She's going to have a terrible life."

"Where else can she go?"

"Nowhere. I know that. But I wish we could do more for her. It's terrible."

"We just can't keep her here indefinitely."

"Why not?"

"Be realistic, Ellie. We're an acute care unit. She used up her coverage months ago. And we're not doing her any favor. The more attached she gets here, the worse it'll be when she leaves."

"How do you know?"

"*Ellie.*"

She laughs. "You always sound so exasperated when you say my name."

"I wonder why," I say.

"I guess I am sort of frustrating sometimes," she says.

My last week on the unit, after two more delays, Tina is finally set to be discharged to a group home. Ellie looks upset that morning at rounds as she presents Tina's case, but she pulls herself together and goes on to her other patients. She just admitted a manic stockbroker, and she presents his case excellently. She'd gotten him medicated within an hour of admission, quieted him down, met with the family — altogether a damn good job.

There's a party that morning at the assistant unit chiefs' meeting — champagne in plastic cups, cheese and crackers, cookies. We assistants all talk about how relieved we are to be finishing, about how we'll finally be able to get to work on our research projects, how we won't be constantly beeped for disasters on the floor, elopements, patients assaulting nurses. It's a nice feeling. We talk about our plans for next year — practice, fellowships, jobs. I'll be at Columbia. I realize I've gotten through it all without any disasters — no suicides, nothing awful. In a few months more, all of residency will be over. Incredible. Even Victor seems relaxed for once.

Later that afternoon, while I'm cleaning out my office, the nurses' station pages me.

"We can't find Ellie," Roberta says. "We need orders on one of her patients. Can you come over?"

"Damn it! Isn't anyone else around?"

"I really think you should come."

I leave the piles of books and journals and case notes spread on the floor and go out to the nurses' station. Everyone's crowded in there, including Roberta and Dr. Blanding and the nurses and the social workers and Ronald and Jan and Lazlo, and when I open the door I see cake and fruit and wine and all that spread out on top of the chart rack.

"Where *is* Ellie?" I say.

No one knows. The party is practically over before Ellie shows up.

"Sorry I'm late," she says. "I've been working on my new admission."

"Did Tina get off all right?"

"Yeah, fine." Ellie seems distracted. She spills wine over the chart rack, and we all back away and throw our paper napkins on the puddle, which drips down over the charts.

"Good job," I say.

"Thanks." She bunches the wet napkins together.

"So now you'll get a new assistant to break in," I say.

"I'm not looking forward to it," she says. "It took me six months to straighten you out."

Her beeper goes off. The record room wants her *stat*.

"Oh damn! I forgot to sign the discharge order," she says. "I'll be right back."

Everyone else scatters, going off to see their last patients of the day. After a while — Ellie's disappeared again — I go back to my office. It's dark by the time I finish moving out.

Studies of the Heart

I

JUST TWENTY MINUTES ago, I was lying in bed, nearly asleep, when I heard my father's footsteps coming up to the attic. I lay there, waiting to see if he was just going to pick up something from his desk. My room, where I moved last January, right after I turned eleven, used to be his study. He still has all his cardiology books here, and piles of medical journals and newspaper clippings, and a door laid across two metal cabinets, and an old wooden desk, and some big blocks of Lucite, with hearts, real *human* hearts, imbedded in them, and a dusty brown medical bag and a brass microscope, and dozens of rubber-banded loops of EKG tapes. Sometimes he comes upstairs late at night to work, and I wake up at two or three in the morning and see him sitting way at the other end of my room, hunched over, reading EKGs or writing on a yellow pad. When I wake up, sometimes he just says hello and tells me to go back to sleep; other times he comes over and sits on my bed and shows me the EKGs, and how you can tell a bundle-branch block from ventricular hypertrophy from an acute myocardial infarction. And sometimes he tells me stories about being in World War II, fighting the Nazis, liberating the concentration camps.

Tonight when he came up, he said, as always, "Are you awake?"

"No," I said. "I'm asleep and this is a dream."

"Such a joker," he said. "You want I should *potch* your *tuchis?*" He sat on the edge of my bed. "What are you doing tomorrow?"

"Nothing," I said. School is out, and camp doesn't start until next week.

"Would you like to come to the hospital?"

"What for?"

"To see a sick patient," he said. "There's an old Negro lady who used to be a maid. She had an acute myocardial infarction two months ago and now has congestive failure."

"And?"

"So she has an arrhythmia. She can't breathe. The Cardiology fellow called up. He doesn't know what to do."

"Give digitalis," I said.

"Very smart," he said. "Are you coming or not? If you're coming, get dressed."

So here I am at the hospital with him, on the Cardiac Unit, while everybody else is home asleep — Mom and Kathy and Jonny and Danny and Susie and little baby Beth and our dog Frisky.

"This is my eldest son," says my father to Mrs. Stefanik, the nurse, a big, red-faced lady who is standing behind the polished wood counter of the nurses' station.

"Nice to meet you," says Mrs. Stefanik. "Are you going to be a famous doctor like your father?"

"Maybe," I say. "Or a baseball player."

Mrs. Stefanik laughs. She offers me a chocolate from a large box. I take one and chew slowly. My father is reading the chart.

Two young doctors in white coats and white pants come over and start talking to my father.

"Oh, hello," one of them says, looking at the white coat I'm wearing, its sleeves rolled up, hem dragging on the floor. "Are you going to be a famous doctor like your father?"

"Looks like he's already started," says the other one.

"He's considering a career in professional sports," my father says.

The two young doctors laugh for only a second, then continue talking in low voices about the patient.

"Have a seat," my father tells me. He leads me to a little alcove to the side of the nurses' station. "Mrs. Stefanik, can you find something for my son to read?"

Mrs. Stefanik brings me some magazines and the box of chocolates, this time insisting that I take two. My father and the two doctors walk down the hall, disappearing.

I wait. I read and read the magazines. I squirm in the chair. My mouth is dry and sweet from the candy. From where I am sitting I can see the ghostly shapes of some beds in the room across the hall, and what I imagine are lumpy blue bodies on them.

Mrs. Stefanik talks on the phone for a while, then goes down the hall and vanishes.

I wait. I am used to waiting, because when there are six kids you always have to wait your turn. But not at this hour of night. Usually when I come here with Dad, he takes me into the patient's room with him, and if it is a nice patient, who doesn't mind, he lifts me up on the bed, and I hold the stethoscope to my ears and listen to the patient's heart sounds: *ka-thunk, ka-thunk, ka-thunk,* sometimes with a *thunk-thunk* thrown in if there's an arrhythmia: *ka-thunk, ka-thunk, thunk-thunk, ka-thunk, ka-thunk.* And the patient shakes my hand and asks if I'm going to be a famous doctor like my father, and isn't it good that I'm getting such an early start?

It is 2:07 in the morning. I have never been up so late at night, except once when Jonny and I stayed up all night to see when it gets light. I am so bored.

Finally Dad and the two young doctors come back. They talk in low voices for a moment, then the two young doctors shake my hand with their moist hands, and Dad says, "So? Time for home?"

We drop off the white coats in his laboratory, then run down six flights — elevators coddle the heart, Dad says — to the front entrance, where the big blue Plymouth is sitting, alone, in the doctors' lot.

At home, we make a snack of cold meatloaf sandwiches on rye with Durkee's sauce and American cheese and pour tall glasses of ice water, and cut a kosher pickle in slices. My father spreads out across the breakfast table, between us, the narrow long tape of an EKG.

A black line wavers along the gridded paper. It rises and falls, occasionally twitching up or down.

"Here it is," he says.

"What?" The pattern before me is confusing, new.

"Fresh off the EKG machine. A very sick patient. See, here the heart stopped —"

"It stopped?"

"For nearly a minute. And here it starts beating again, after we gave her a shot of . . ."

I look at my father in surprise. It's the woman we just saw.

"Is she going to live?" I ask.

"Tonight she almost died."

"But is she going to *live?*" I look for clues in the gridded tape.

"This may be her last night," he says.

I finish my sandwich, there in the yellow breakfast room, looking out the dark windows at the ghostly trunk of the apple tree outside, and beyond it, across the lawn, at the picket fence that separates our lawn from the Rineharts', and beyond that, at the dark bulk of what, in the daytime, must just be houses, walls, porches, garages, but which now seems to pulse with life.

"Bedtime," my father says.

I stand.

"Clean off your place," he says. "Don't leave a mess for your mother."

I I

It is a beautiful Saturday morning, perfect for driving in the country — cool, still misty under the trees, and there aren't many cars out yet, just some pickup trucks full of pumpkins and corn and logs that whiz by us. We are in the white Corvair, heading east, past Richmond and Chagrin and County Line Road. My little brother Jonny and I are sitting in the front seat next to Dad, and in the back seat are metal boxes with his research equipment.

We suddenly swerve out across the yellow line, to pass a black carriage being pulled by a horse. My brother goes wild. "What's that? What's that?" he asks.

"It's just the Amish," I say.

We go up and down little hills. Jonny says he is carsick.

"Just take deep breaths," I advise. "Anyway, we're almost there."

We're in farm country now: corn, cows, barns, parachutes.

"I see one!"

"Where?" says Jonny.

"There!"

"Where? I don't see."

"It's red and white. See, it's falling down."

"Hold still," our father says. We turn onto a dirt road, bumping along it, then turn across the field, dodging a big hole filled with rocks and rusty metal, and drive like crazy, raising dust, to the very edge of the woods, where a dozen cars are parked around a big, old, green school bus.

"Where's the plane?" I say. I bump my chin on the dash-board, looking. I see the plane. I see the plane. I open the door, run out, looking in the air. A second, a third, a fourth parachute have appeared. The red and white parachute is coming down to the ground, a man hanging below. He angles down to the ground, does a quick somersault as he hits, and comes up on his feet, red and white nylon billowing around him.

"It's Will," my father announces. We run with him over to the parachute. Will, a tall, thin man, is wearing an orange jumpsuit. He balls up the parachute material in his arms to stop it from catching the wind. He is standing, I see as we approach, in the middle of a white circle, drawn with chalk. There is another, larger circle in which we are standing.

"They're coming down," says Jonny. He's scared.

"Dad, we have to move," I say.

Dad is talking to Will about the research study. Today he wants to go up in the plane. He needs blood samples in the air, before they jump, to measure how the heart gets ready.

The other parachutes swirl above up in the blue sky, one red and yellow, the other two green and white. They are swirling around, coming down on us. Dad yells at us to get over to the car.

We run to the side of the field, by the old school bus. Our father is still in the middle of the circle, with Will.

"He's going to get hit," Jonny says. But the wind has blown the parachutists to the edge of the field, over by the road.

"Look at that. That one almost got run over," I tell Jonny. Today I am in a mood to scare him. "If the wind blows the wrong way you can get killed," I say.

"No you can't," my brother says.

"Oh yeah?" I turn him around, and point out what is in the trees.

"That's nothing. That's just a kite."

"That's a parachute," I say. "See, it's red and blue. Last week the wind blew the wrong way and somebody came down right there."

"Was he all right?"

"No, he died. He was torn into little pieces."

We walk around the bus, over to where a big machine sits on the ground, throbbing.

"That's a generator," I tell Jonny. "It makes electricity."

"What do you make it out of?" Jonny asks. "Did he *really* die?"

The plane is coming down lower, low over the barn and farmhouse, so it looks as if it will crash into them. Then it glides down onto the field, bumping over the furrows, and finally comes to a stop near the chalk circles.

I reach into the back seat of the Corvair for one of the metal boxes.

"Sometimes the plane crashes, too," I say.

He's hanging on my every word, but I can tell he doesn't believe me. The metal box bangs against my side as we walk across the field toward the plane. The door on the side of the plane is open, and some men with parachutes on their backs are going inside. Our father is leaning on the wing.

"See that hole in the ground?" I say.

"Where?" says Jonny.

"Over there. You know what happened last week?"

"What?"

"One of the parachutes got caught in the propeller and the plane came crashing down on the ground."

"No it didn't," Jonny says, but there is a question in his voice.

"Sure it did." I hand my father the metal box. He takes out a stethoscope and blood pressure cuff and looks inside at the syringes and test tubes and bottles of alcohol and the cotton balls, to make sure everything is there.

"Watch out for your brother," he says. He gets into the plane.

"Okay," I say.

The men pull the door closed.

"It did not," he says.

We back away.

"Oh yeah?" I say. "Why else is there that hole in the ground?"

The plane takes off, bumping across the field. I hold my brother's hand. We wait for our father to come down.

I I I

Sometimes my father comes up to the attic and tells stories. He tells the story of how his mother's brother was kicked in the stomach by some hoods, criminals, in Poland, and how something burst inside and he died. He tells of Dillonvale, Ohio, where his mother and father settled after they left Poland, and where his father opened a store with his partner, Hellerstein and Finkelstein, Outfitters from Head to Foot. He tells what it was like when the coalminers went out on strike and scabs were sent down from Chicago, carrying guns. He tells about the swinging bridge over the creek, which he was afraid he'd fall off every time he crossed it. He tells about being the smallest boy in the class. He tells about his family moving to Cleveland during the Depression. He tells about medical school and joining the army, and the war. Those are the best stories, the war stories.

When my friend Ron comes over to spend the night, we always ask my father to tell war stories. He tells us how two of his jeep drivers were killed right next to him. He tells how he was wounded. He tells how he pulled men out of burning tanks. He tells how they liberated the concentration camps and found thousands of starving people. He tells how he was captured by the Russians outside Berlin, in the closing days of the war, and was mistaken for a German spy. Really? we say. Is that really true? We lie awake late at night, talking about guns and tanks and bombers, and what we'd do if the Nazis came and tried to take us away.

And in the afternoons, when I get tired of reading, sitting in my orange reclining chair at the end of my room, near the window, I set down my *Superman* comic or *Tom Swift* book and begin looking through my father's things. In the closet are large, crackly bags full of old army clothes, green wool coats and khaki jackets with silver and gold bars still attached to their shoulders, and dusty old army boots, and three bayonets in sheaths, and a bulky white sheepskin coat, fleece turned in, which my father took from a German prisoner, and piles of German books, and a framed steel relief of a half-naked woman raising her arm before a crowd of soldiers, with a banner fluttering overhead that reads DEUTSCHLAND ÜBER ALLES. My father broke off the woman's arm when he took the relief from a German house, and now the arm dangles from its shoulder by a chain. One day, looking in the back drawers of his wooden desk, I find a canvas bag inside which are letters, small trophies and medals, photographs — tiny photographs showing piles of starved, dead bodies at a concentration camp. Scared, oddly excited, I fit everything back into the bag and hide it in the drawer, swearing that my father's secrets will be safe with me.

I read and reread comics from the pile beside my chair. My hero is Superman. My father reads my comics, too, three or four at a time. He takes them downstairs and reads them at the breakfast table.

"I want to keep up with what you're reading," he says.

One night my father comes up to my room while I am sleeping.

"Are you awake?" he says.

"What?" I say drowsily.

"No lights," he says. I lie back. "Listen," he says. "This is no joke. The world is about to be destroyed."

"When?" I say at last.

"Tonight," he says. He tells me to listen carefully. I shouldn't be scared. He has a plan.

I sit up, leaning forward as he talks.

It's absurd, his plan, but as he tells it to me I find myself wanting to believe it, somehow hoping that it could just be true. What he says is that there is a rocket in the basement, which he has been building ever since he found out that the world was going to be destroyed, a rocket that is just big enough for one person. What he wants me to do is to go downstairs with him. It's time for me to go.

I get out of bed, put on my slippers, and follow him down the creaky stairs to the second floor, where everyone is sleeping. We go from room to room, from Jonny to Danny to Kathy to Susie to Beth, and in each room I whisper goodbye. Then, excited, terrified, clinging to the banister in the darkness, I follow him downstairs to the first floor.

"Shh," he says.

We stand in the hallway, in the darkness, before the dimly glowing panels of the front door. He leads me into the living room and stops abruptly. There we wait, between the dim white outline of the couch and the back windows, which are half shrouded with curtains, and through which I can see the back yard, the apple tree, and beyond it, the rose trellises and the brick wall. All of this, I realize with a thrill, is about to be destroyed. I wonder what the rocket looks like, and how comfortable it will be, and how long I'll be in space before I land on a new planet, and what that wonderful new world will be like, and exactly what superpowers I'll have.

"Okay," my father says at last. "That's that."

"What?" I ask.

"It won't be tonight," he replies.

"What won't?"

"The world won't be destroyed after all."

"Oh," I say, disappointed beyond all words. "What about the rocket?"

"Another time," he says. He begins walking out of the living room, toward the hallway. Eventually, I follow him back upstairs.

I V

The first day of Cardiovascular Surgery rotation, I show up in the ICU at 5:00 A.M. The ICU is an enormous crevasse of linoleum and glass, sealed off from the rest of the hospital. The nurses' station is in the middle and patient rooms are on the perimeter, behind sliding glass doors. It's cold. It feels as if a wind is blowing constantly, starting from the floor and going up through the ceiling. Shivering, I sit in the nurses' station, drinking coffee, until the rest of the team shows up at 5:45.

Raklov, a thin, exhausted-looking man in rumpled greens and a white coat that looks like it's been slept in for weeks, is the chief resident. He introduces me to the interns and residents on the team, and we begin rounds. We go through sliding doors into the chilly, windy patient rooms. The patients have tubes, connected to suction machines in the wall, coming out of their chests. Some are on respirators. A few have odd, sleek machines at the foot of their beds, machines that thump every few seconds. Intra-aortic balloon pumps, one of the interns tells me. The cold air is from a laminar flow exhaust system, such as you have in a chemistry lab.

We go off the unit to the ward, where the patients go when they are stable. We look at chest wounds, removing and replacing gauze pads, seeing how the long gash from the base of the neck to the solar plexus is healing, whether there is pain or swelling, whether suture material is showing through. The patients complain of pain, but they look happy, relieved, and they're up, sitting on the edge of their beds or taking a few steps in the hall.

Our team has two cases today, Raklov says.

We go into the locker room and change into greens, put on masks and caps and shoe covers, and push through into the surgery suite. We stand before scrub sinks, washing our hands and arms up above the elbows with plastic pads full of yellow soap. We scrub our hands with the soft bristles on one side of the pad, rinse our arms and turn off the water with foot pedals, and back into the operating room, water dripping off our arms. We dry our arms with sterile towels, and the nurses hold up gowns for us so we can slide into them, arms first, and they tie them around us, and they pull long plastic gloves over our hands.

We turn to the table. The patient is already out, and the anesthesiologist is securing the tube in his throat. Raklov motions to me to get out of the way so he and Berg, the intern, can put cloth drapes over the patient's body, keeping his chest and left leg exposed, and then unfold a paper drape with a "window" in it over his chest. The attending, Dr. Wharton, has come in and gowned up.

We stand at the table. The nurse adjusts a tray of instruments over the foot of the bed. Raklov stands over the patient's bare leg.

"Scalpel," says Dr. Wharton.

Wharton feels for landmarks on the chest. He begins to cut — a smooth slice opening up the skin from the V at the base of the neck to the tail of the xyphoid, the lower end of the sternum. Raklov blots away blood with gauze pads, and bovies one or two blood vessels that are still bleeding.

"Saw," says Dr. Wharton.

The nurse hands over something that looks like a high-tech version of a Black and Decker tool. Dr. Wharton slides the tip of it under the upper edge of the patient's sternum and begins cutting downward, until he reaches the end of the incision. Then there is something for me to do: to hold the side of the chest back with a retractor, so Dr. Wharton and Dr. Raklov can go through the pericardium.

And there is the heart. Beating against the retractor, bulging up every second, red as a newborn baby's head, shrinking back down inside. Dr. Wharton lifts, clamps, slices, sticks a tube in an open vessel, sutures, cuts, tells Raklov to move in. Raklov holds, clamps, cuts, suctions, then holds a tube in his hand. I watch, thinking of the day my father called three years ago, after his heart surgery, how I was sitting in my dorm room that day and the phone rang and he said, Are you there? and I said yes and he said listen carefully, I'm in the hospital, I've had surgery, and then went on to describe in great, woozy detail — his voice fading every minute or two — how the pain had come on in his office, how he knew what it was and called the Surgery suite, and said to them, I have a patient to schedule for a coronary bypass, and they said who is the patient and he said, it is I; and how odd that seemed to me at the time, hearing about it a week afterward, and how I thought then, do I really want to be a doctor? And how there was an interruption and somebody said that was enough, and then he said he had to go, and that his chest hurt, not his heart, I was to understand, but the incision, which pain, though non-lethal, was nevertheless more than he could take. And how I thought suddenly, he wants me to be just like him, he wants to live his life over again through me, that's why he wants me to be a cardiologist and researcher. And how ashamed I felt for being absolutely furious at him, which I knew I just shouldn't be.

"Hold this," Raklov says, pushing in my direction a plastic tube that extends down through the aorta, into the heart. I reach for the tube, around Dr. Wharton's hand and Raklov's hand, and Raklov lets go of the tube, and then the tube is drifting upward, out of both our hands. We both grab for it; Raklov gets it first, and holds it before me.

"You *got* it?" he says.

"Got it," I say.

"Let me see that for a second," Dr. Wharton says. "Did I see an air bubble go in there?" He clamps the tube near the aorta and taps the side of it with a probe. "I should have told you to hold it down," he says.

We do two more bypasses that day, and two more the next, then a valve replacement, and an experimental balloon dilation procedure. I find I really love cardiac surgery, and Dr. Wharton and Dr. Raklov let me do more of the cutting and suturing, and even some blunt dissection in the chest. I'm one of the best medical students they've ever had on the service, Berg says. I consider a career in surgery. Would I like it, getting up at five every morning, coming home at midnight, having the unequaled privilege of cutting the human heart?

One day, while we're on rounds, a middle-aged woman comes up to us, hysterical.

"I brought a whole man in here," she says. "Now look what I have — half a man!"

She points at her husband, who is lying in bed; he had a stroke during the operation and is paralyzed on one side. That happens sometimes. One of the nurses has to go over to her and calm her down. We continue on rounds. It's not until that night, when I'm on my way out of the Med Center, that the thought strikes me that it might have been my fault. I go back along the long corridors to the ward and, backpack over my shoulder, lean over the chart rack, looking for the right chart, the chart of the half-man. I look around. Is anyone watching me, here at eight at night in the nurses' station?

Was it I? I leaf through the chart, looking at admission notes, medication records, vital signs. I get the order book off the cart by the elevator, just in case there was some mistake, and look to see whether it was I. It wasn't. The operation was done two days before I came on service. But all the way home, riding my bicycle on a path through eucalyptus trees, all I can think of is that tube wiggling free, and think, I did it, I did it, despite irrefutable evidence to the contrary.

V

So the other day my father calls. Actually, my mother calls and talks to me first and then yells for him to come down from the study and hands the phone to him because he was really the one who wanted to talk to me but she had to, I guess, warm me up. So we talk. What's going on here and what's going on there and about all the various brothers and sisters and what's going on with them, all the usual stuff, and what I'm doing next year, now that residency is finally almost over — twenty-fifth grade, we always joke. I tell him how I've been rushing all over the city interviewing for jobs, how I've finally decided to take a fellowship in public psychiatry, working with chronic patients. Does that lead anywhere? he says. And there's the inevitable question, as though nothing else counts, am I doing any research? Yes, I say, and for the first time in my life it's true. I am doing research despite vigorous, intense, at times frenzied efforts to avoid it; yes, eventually, everybody here has to do research. And where will you live next year, he says. I tell him. We go through all the details. That's a lot of money, he says. This is New York, I say. It's a bargain. Here you could have a house and two acres and a swimming pool for that, he says. I'm sure you could, I say, but then you wouldn't be in New York, would you? And what are *your* plans? I say. Oh, he says, in the same tone as that day when he called after his heart surgery, I really don't know. You don't, I say. What are the possibilities? And he talks about the possibilities and for a few moments it's as though I'm the father and he's the son and in some peculiar way he wants me to give him advice the same way he always wants me to want him to give me advice, which I always pretend to do but end up feeling angry about afterward because I don't feel listened to, but then I realize I'm not listening, either, so I listen. When he's seventy he will have to give up his laboratory, he says. I guess that will be hard, I say. Yes, he says. He could go to another hospital, he says, or he could go into practice for a lot of money, or he could just go down to Florida and lie in the sun. That doesn't sound like you, I say. No it doesn't, does it, he says, but I have to give up the laboratory, and for a moment it's as though he's ten years old. And then my wife, who has been watching TV, gets up and says, Hey, if we're going swimming we have to leave now; the pool closes in forty-five minutes. So I say, Hey, Dad, I have to go in a . . . And he says, I don't want to keep you. Click.

And before I know it he's gone.

NOTES

NOTES

Page 14. Gale, Robert P. "Advances in the Treatment of Acute Myelogenous Leukemia." *New England Journal of Medicine* 300:21 (1979), pp. 1189–99.

Page 20. Sontag, Susan. *Illness as Metaphor.* New York: Farrar, Straus & Giroux, 1978, pp. 65–70.

Page 83. Williams, William Carlos. *Selected Poems.* New York: New Directions, 1969, pp. 94–96.

Page 90. Trilling, Lionel, ed. *The Selected Letters of John Keats.* New York: Farrar, Straus and Young, 1951, pp. 146–67.

Page 105. Lazarus, J. Michael. "Complications in Hemodialysis: An Overview." *Kidney International* 18 (1980), pp. 783–96.

Pages 125, 133. Foucault, Michel. *The Birth of the Clinic: An Archaeology of Medical Perception.* New York: Pantheon Books, 1973, pp. 124–48.

ABOUT THE AUTHOR

A graduate of Harvard University, David Hellerstein received his medical degree from Stanford University Medical School in 1980. His writing has appeared in *Esquire, Ms., Harper's, North American Review, Science Digest,* and other national publications. He was awarded the Pushcart Prize for Best Essay in 1980, and a Mac-Dowell Fellowship in 1984. At present, David Hellerstein practices psychiatry in New York, where he lives with his wife. He has recently completed his first novel.